The Biohacking Manifesto

The scientific blueprint for a long, healthy and happy life using cutting edge anti-aging and neuroscience based hacks

James Lee

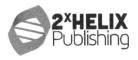

2ˣHELIX
Publishing

Important Disclaimer

Contents

Introduction

This book emerged out of just a few reader emails suggesting that I release a compendium of three of my most popular books – The Methuselah Project, Your Brain Electric and Brain Hacks. However rather than just cobble these three books together, slap a new cover and title on, then take a Scrooge McDuck bath in all the money that selling $6.99 eBooks brings[1], I thought I would take the opportunity to revisit some of the science to dig up some genuinely new and interesting content.

What exactly *is* "biohacking" you may ask?

Biohacking is just a fancy word for using science-based tools and shortcuts for optimising your own biological potential. This can enable you to –

- Maximise longevity and life span

- Optimise memory and cognitive function using little-known nootropic supplements and drugs

- Optimise your own neurochemistry to maximise happiness and well-being

- Improve physical performance and underlying physiological health

- Prevent and repair premature cellular aging

The field I cover moves quickly. Two years ago I was recommending resveratrol to all and sundry, however the most recent research has shown that, until we are able to create a more potent and bioavailable form, we should save our cash for more effective longevity-promoting agents.

However it is arguable the area of nootropics which is evolving the quickest. This is not surprising, as this is an area of cognitive neuroscience and pharmacology which prides itself for sitting at the cutting edge. If something doesn't work and the trials are inconclusive, you will soon hear about it on the /r/nootropics sub-Reddit or the Longecity Brain Health forum.

I am pleased to report that the resultant book you are about to read forms one of the most comprehensive biohacking manuals available anywhere, looking at three of the main pillars of this area of study – anti-aging, mood support and nootropics.

As with all my guides, my commitment to you the dear reader, is to continually update the content as the science evolves. One of the core tenets of solid science is to be prepared to change your position if the scientific consensus changes or new studies emerge with conflicting findings. As anyone who has been reading my books since I started will know, I am never embarrassed to admit I was wrong or change my view. I will continue to honour this.

In Part 1 I look at the science of anti-aging and the various ways in which we can

---

[1] I am being facetious by the way. My eBook income wouldn't permit even the shallowest of baths, even if I converted it to pennies.

harness our understanding to promote longevity. In Part 2 I provide a comprehensive guidebook on the fundamentals of neurochemistry and how we can use this information to generate diagnostic tools along with ways we can hack our neurochemistry. Then finally, in Part 3, I outline the various agents we have at our disposal for turbo-charging memory and cognitive processes.

It is important to point out that the arenas of longevity promotion, neurochemistry and brain enhancement will have natural overlap. My first instinct was to search and destroy any duplication to achieve my beloved tight page count. However in the end I have decided to leave much of the original content as is. Repetition is vital for comprehension. The more times you read the same piece of information, the more likely it will be to stick. So there are multiple times throughout this book where you will read about things like omega 3, curcumin and astaxanthin. This is not surprising considering the virtually globally beneficial effects substances such as these have on the human body and brain.

There is nothing in this book that will cure cancer or turn you into a superhero. What there is however, is a range of pharmacological and non-pharmacological tools to enable you to get an edge over the general population.

Information is power and you are holding power in your hands at this very moment.

James Lee

May 2015

Part 1 – Anti-Aging and Longevity

The human obsession with long life and immortality predates even the mythical *Fountain of Youth*, which was a mythical spring thought to bestow immortality on whomever drank from it or bathed in it. Spanish explorer Juan Ponce de León reputedly stumbled on what would become modern day Florida while searching for it in the 1600s. Even before this, the Fountain of Youth was referred to in the writings Herodotus some legends surrounding Alexander the Great. Likewise, the *Elixir of Life* mentioned in Chinese, Indian and European mythology reportedly confers similar benefits to whoever should be fortunate enough to drink it.

However, surely in mythology the undisputed king of long life must be Methuselah, who *reportedly* (and I use that term loosely) lived to the ripe old age of 969. Many scholars quite soberly reject this claim, saying that his actual age was either mistranslated (and was actually closer to 96.9 years old) or that the story is not meant to be taken literally. Taking a moment to imagine what it would be like to live to 969 is actually quite helpful because most people assume they would choose immortality if they had the choice. When you start to imagine each 50 year block, you realize why the finite human lifespan is actually a great gift. I can't imagine what Methuselah would have done to occupy himself for all those years besides woodworking and shooing teenagers off his lawn. *Matlock* didn't start showing on TV until the 1980s, well after Methuselah died, so it is hard to imagine how he spent his evenings.

In modern times, this same basic desire to live as long as possible has led to the science of anti-aging, which is dedicated to extending lifespan and making these additional years happy and productive. After all, it would be pointless to live until 150 years of age if you are forced to endure those last 50 years bedridden, with just a faint pulse signaling to relatives and those hoping to be included in your will, that you are indeed, actually still alive.

When people think of anti-aging, they think of oxidative stress, antioxidants, expensive face creams and the like. However this is far too narrow a definition for anti-aging as I see it. I prefer to use the term *life-extension* or even *longevity-promotion*, which is more descriptive of what it is I am looking to achieve with this book.

Life extension is not just about eating broccoli and lathering *Crème de la Mer* on your face each night. It's also about playing the odds. Each poor decision you make regarding your health accumulates. For example, imagine that you smoke a pack a day of cigarettes ever each, drink a six pack of beer each night, drink a liter of Coca Cola each day while you work, take cocaine on weekends with your buddies, ride a high-powered motorbike everywhere (sometimes without a helmet), go skydiving each weekend, surf in an area notorious for great white sharks, have a high-stress job, rarely eat fruit or vegetables and eat a diet based primarily around junk food.

Sometimes this is referred to as additive risk, because each additional high-risk activity adds risk to life and limb. This is why those soundbites comparing your risk of dying from a high risk activity (such as surfing in shark-infested waters) to the risk of dying in your car on the way to work are pointless. One of these risks is relatively unavoidable.

It is up to you how many of these risks you want to add to your life, without resorting to living as a kind of bubble-boy, afraid of anything remotely pleasurable.

How long do you think you will live? Each of your poor diet and lifestyle choices is like playing a game of Russian roulette. One day there will be a bullet in the chamber. So life extension is about a holistic plan that incrementally decreases your odds of dying by misadventure or developing a preventable disease. This is all about reducing risk, not about guaranteeing anything. Sometimes people can become fatalistic when they hear of the health fanatic that dropped dead at 40 with a heart attack. *If it can happen to that guy, why bother?*

There are always going to be exceptions and people with certain genetic issues that may predispose them to particular problems. However the fact remains that if you make good choices, take good care of yourself and follow some basic nutritional and supplemental principles, you will dramatically increase your odds of making it to 100 and beyond.

Some researchers have more ambitious targets, believing that we have a potential maximum life span of 150 years or more. Some even believe there is no theoretical maximum and if they crack the code we could live indefinitely.

Me personally, I would be comfortable with 100. I think that by the time I reach that age, I will be well and truly ready to throw in the towel and move on to whatever awaits me on the other side, if anything.

You are holding in your hand a guide to getting to whatever your personal target age may be. Firstly I want to give you some of the science that underpins the concept of aging and what we can do to work around some of the impediments to a long and healthy life. Then I will go through some of the practical steps you can take to get you where you want to go.

Originally, aging was viewed as the natural process of wear and tear your body goes through as it fights the *second law of thermodynamics*. The second law of thermodynamics refers to a range of universal concepts, including the fact that heat will transfer from warmer to cooler areas over time, leading to equal temperatures. This is why a glass of water left at room temperature will eventually move towards whatever the ambient temperature is (all other things being equal). However the second law of thermodynamics also states that compound, ordered bodies (anything with mass) in a closed system will gradually move towards disorder. This is often misconstrued to refer to processes such as the decay of a dead body or a piece of wood rotting in the ground. So originally, aging was viewed as your body moving inexorably towards disorder, and when it reached a particular tipping point (through damage or whatever mechanism), death would occur.

However the problem with all this "second law of thermodynamics" talk is that it wasn't actually correct. The aging of the human body has nothing to do with the second law because the human body isn't a closed system. Your body is constantly taking in energy and nutrients from your environment for metabolic functions and general repair – it doesn't operate in a vacuum.

Let me use an analogy – Say you are made of building blocks that look just like the blocks little babies use to build things, and next to you is an inexhaustible pile of replacement blocks. Each time one of your blocks breaks, you can just grab a new block and slide it into place just where the old, broken one had been. In this scenario, you would not be breaking the second law by continuing to exist in perpetuity.

Similarly, sometime in the 19th century, this idea that aging was an unavoidable consequence of the second law was discredited and abandoned. Well not entirely. The second law is to this day sometimes misappropriated in Creationist circles as a means to explain why evolution violates this fundamental principle of the universe, with *intelligent design* is the only logical explanation.

This is an exciting concept to ponder. Due to the fact that animals are constantly swapping energy and other "stuff" with their environment, there is no theoretical reason why humans or other animals could not achieve immortality. However, clearly when you think about it, immortality would, on balance be a terrible idea for just about every living creature on earth. Which is why biology appears to have put in place a range of self-destruct mechanisms designed to keep populations of animals young, strong and healthy. Unburdened by a large population of elderly specimens.

Despite the fact that this process is occurring essentially from birth (or some may say, from early adulthood when growing has stopped and decay starts to accelerate), aging generally becomes noticeable only from middle age as things start to malfunction and break. Another way to look at this is that your body undergoes constant repair and regeneration work throughout life. However, as you age, slowly your body starts struggling to keep up with this repair work. It is thought that certain types of cancers start in this way. Researchers believe that quite regularly, certain cells mutate and become potentially cancerous, however they are quickly eliminated by your immune system. As you age, these mutations increase, making it harder for your immune system to keep up and more likely that one of these mutant cells will be missed – leading to cancer.

However it is not purely environmental aging at work, but also a complex interaction between your genetics and your environment. In the past, people often referred to "nature versus nurture", which was basically referring to genes and environment. Was someone born that way or did something happen to them that triggered a certain illness or behavior? However nowadays as science has progressed, the buzz word has become epigenetics, which basically refers to your genes and how they can be turned on or off by your environment. Let me give the example of a smoker. Why is it that some people can smoke a pack a day for life and never get lung cancer while others are struck down in midlife, despite smoking the same amount of cigarettes? This is because a small minority of smokers have a particular genetic makeup that prevents them from developing lung cancer. I should point out an important point however – many smokers point to these rare outliers who don't get cancer as a reason why it doesn't matter whether you smoke or not. However this is a complete fallacy. Not only are these people exceedingly rare, this belief doesn't take epigenetics into account. You should never base your beliefs and decisions on the visible minority (they are the visible minority because most of the other long-term smokers are not particularly visible unless you are a "*Long Island medium*")

So any scientific research aimed at extending the life span of humans must also look at genetics, not just environmental aging. As Danica Chen, UC Berkeley's assistant professor of Nutritional Science and Toxicology states *"A major goal of the aging field is to utilize knowledge of genetic regulation to treat age-related diseases."*

In a nutshell, irrespective of whether we are looking at genetics or environmental aging, anti-aging research is focused on slowing down, inhibiting or reversing the process of aging to increase the human life span.

There is also a philosophical debate in scientific fields as to whether the aging process should be viewed as a disease or a natural process. Harvard Medical School's David Sinclair says *"I don't see aging as a disease, but as a collection of quite predictable diseases caused by the deterioration of the body".* In contrast, David Gems, Assistant Director of the Institute of Healthy Aging, believes that aging must be considered as a form of disease. However irrespective of the philosophy underpinning the science, the fact remains that all researchers are united in their ambition to both extend the human life span and make any extra years pleasant and disability free for as many people as possible. And coming out of this work over the past two decades has been some amazing advances in our understanding of the process of aging and potential ways in which these processes can be modulated.

Aging is a complicated process that includes a range of parameters health, cognitive function, and level of physical mobility. Who is actually older – the 80 year old who can run a marathon and write a novel or a 30 year old with type-2 diabetes that sits on the couch all day because of a bad back and muscle soreness? As part of this thinking we need to broaden our definition of anti-aging far beyond the concept of life-extension. I think a better target would be *"life-extension + life-optimization"*.

Despite this, some researchers believe that by targeting one, you naturally target the other. The latest issue of the *Public Policy & Aging Report (PP&AR)*, titled *The Longevity Dividend: Geroscience Meets Geropolitics,* states that the best way to achieve improved longevity and quality of life is by targeting the slowing down of the process of biological aging rather than targeting the individual diseases separately.

Life expectancy and life span

It is when we look at life expectancy rather than life span that we can see why the definition of anti-aging needs to be expanded away from narrow areas of focus such as oxidative stress. In 2002, scientists pointed out that life expectancy is has been on a continuous upward trend for the past 160 years, with life expectancy increasing by a quarter of a year annually. This average life-expectancy (defined as the average number of years a person will live) - has increased from 46 years at the start of the 20th century to 65 years today. However, the irrefutable fact during the same period is that the maximum potential lifespan hasn't changed in that whole time. Not only does this call into question our ability to extend this maximum lifespan (at the time of writing the oldest person to have lived – and been verified – so Methuselah doesn't count - was France's Jeanne Calment, who lived to 122), but also points to the important point I made earlier – life-expectancy is determined by a range of factors, not just chronological aging. In the last hundred years or so, the biggest driver of increased life expectancy by far has been our ability to treat infectious diseases which were previously often fatal. Some awful diseases (such as smallpox), have been virtually wiped off the planet. When you stop to ponder this you realize that any effort to extend your own personal lifespan to 100 and beyond (with your physical health and faculties intact) must tackle the problem from multiple angles, not just slowing down chronological aging.

So while we will continue to see increases in life expectancy (particularly in the area of cancer research and improvements in our understanding of heart disease), until a truly major breakthrough is made, any improvements on our maximum life span will only ever be incremental. Put another way, as lifestyle and medical care continues to improve, more people with "longevity-friendly" genes will survive long enough to seriously challenge Jeanne Calment's record.

However don't give up hope. After all, at various times over the past few decades certain scientists have claimed that we would not see any more improvements in life expectancy. Yet we continue to see improvements each year, little by little. So while I can't see anything on the near horizon that would extend life span much beyond current levels, I could be proven wrong with a single major discovery or development.

Nevertheless, the focus of this book will be on increasing your own personal life expectancy, not your maximum life span. If someone promises to help you live to 130, don't hand over any money!

In terms of life expectancy, Japan remains the clear front-runner among major countries with a large enough sample size (Smaller locations such as - Monaco with an average life expectancy of 89.63 years and Macau with 84.46 years don't have a big enough sample size to draw sweeping conclusions). A Japanese person today can expect to reach the fulsome age of 84. In fact, in Japan alone there are more than 50,000 centenarians (those aged 100 years and above). This contrasts with countries like Chad, which have a disappointingly low life expectancy of 49.07 years. Curiously, not far from Chad, an Ethiopian farmer by the name of Dhaqabo Ebba has claimed to be over 160 years old. Ebba, who is, unsurprisingly, retired, has apparently lived through and witnessed a *"transfer of power among all of the five Gadaa Oromo political parties in four rotations"*, which would put his age at over 160. As he doesn't possess a birth certificate, scientists are currently working on verifying his age by other means. If his age is confirmed as being 160 years old, I will start getting my knife and fork, along with various condiments ready to consume my own hat.

Increases in life expectancy are now even capturing the attention of mainstream press, as evidenced by this article in the UK's *Guardian Newspaper* which said *""Every minute that you spend reading this article, the average life expectancy in Britain will rise by 12 seconds. By the time you finish reading, your life expectancy will have gone up by six minutes. This time tomorrow, it will have increased by almost five hours. The reason is clear: rapid advances in medicine and biology have been one of the biggest achievements of the past century and we are all living longer. Where anyone reaching the age of 60 was considered to be near death's door at the turn of the 20th century, it is barely old enough for retirement at the turn of the 21st century."* [14]

So, if the science is advancing so impressively, the next question must logically be – *What causes biological aging?*

Why and how do we age?

There are a massive number of theories on why and how we age. Many of these are not "either or" theories either, with their being a strong likelihood that the answer turns out to be a combination of factors. For example, it is highly likely that telomere shortening plays a role, along with oxidative stress also. However, broadly speaking, we can break the theories into two main groups –

1. "Programmed senescence" style theories – These theories say that we have an upper limit to our life span that is built into our genetics

2. "Damage" theories – These theories say that aging is caused by a range of changes caused by environmental damage. This damage can be "wear and tear" style damage or damage from genetic mutation caused by faulty repair processes.

According to programmed senescence style theories, aging is driven by an innate internal clock that is controlled by gene expression. Usually this internal clock is represented by telomeres, which sit at the end of chromosomes. Telomeres have been found to gradually shorten as an animal ages and this has been used as an example of how we have an internal process driving the aging process. However even this theory gets complicated due to the fact that many scientists believe that oxidative stress accelerates the process of telomere shortening.

Under these types of theories, any advances in longevity will require some form of modulation of this internal clock by, for example, slowing down telomere shortening somehow.

Under damage-style theories, it is believed that aging is caused by a range of processes which damage an organism. The organism either can't keep up its internal repair work or the repair work is faulty, leading to genetic mutations such as cancer. Two of the most commonly mentioned drivers of environmental aging are oxidative stress and inflammation. However there are a multitude of similar theories which could also be involved to some extent. For example, there is a theory linking life span with basal metabolic rate that proposes an inverse relationship between an animal's metabolic rate and how long it can possibly live for. So, under this theory, elephants would live a long time and hummingbirds much less so. This is probably one of the oldest theories as to why we age, being first proposed more than a century ago.

Now, before we move on to exactly *how* to slow down the aging process, let's familiarize ourselves with some of the core concepts and theories of aging in detail.

Senescence

At the cellular level, senescence refers to the point at which a cell ceases to divide. Based on experiments *in vitro* (in a test tube essentially), cells appear to have around 50 divisions before they become senescent and no longer divide. This upper limit to the number of divisions is known as the *Hayflick limit*. These senescent cells then just hang around, continuing to do their job until they are destroyed by other events (think of it as dying of natural causes). It is believed that these senescent cells hold one of the key clues to the aging process. In certain animal tests, removing senescent cells led to various improvements in age related conditions.

However, at various points during a cell's period of dividing (before reaching the *Hayflick limit*), certain external shocks or sudden damage can trigger a process known as apoptosis – programmed cell death. When a cell is damaged, attempts are made to repair the cell so it can continue to function. However in certain cases where the body decides that the damage is too great, it will trigger apoptosis and exterminate the cell.

The concept of senescence and apoptosis is central to any theory of aging because it touches on one of the great paradoxes of aging. You have probably read about apoptosis and senescence and thought - *Great! So why don't we just turn off this programmed cell death, allowing us to become immortal?* Well, there is one big problem – cancer. This is exactly what happens when apoptosis is switched off. At the cellular level, cancer begins when a cell suddenly decides that it won't commit cellular suicide and decides that rapid division instead is more its scene. This happens quite regularly however usually these cells are immediately identified and dealt with swiftly and without mercy. However, when the immune system is compromised or overloaded with these cells, that's when cancer has the chance to grow and spread.

This is why any tinkering with senescence and apoptosis needs to be done with extreme caution to ensure that cancer isn't the end result. Where this research gets truly interesting is in the studies of animals that do not appear to experience measurable senescence and do not appear to get cancer. The humble lobster is one example of this. Immortality, or served on a plate with *Mornay* sauce – there's no middle ground.

The equal and opposite of cancer is an accelerated aging disease such as *progeria*, where young children have tragically aged at such a dramatic rate that they look like elderly people. Any study of aging and related cancers could benefit from a deeper understanding of what drives these kinds of accelerated aging diseases.

A possible mechanism by which to clear out senescent cells and other cellular waste to slow down the aging process could be to optimize the natural process of *autophagy*. Autophagy is a process that keeps everything humming along nicely at the cellular level, preventing further damage that could come from harmful debris left floating around.

Not surprisingly, scientists have found that modulating the process of autophagy appears to trigger an anti-aging effect. The most promising example of this is in the area of caloric restriction for life extension. As of today, caloric restriction is arguably the single most potent and measurable life-extending technique we have at our disposal. A few years ago scientists noticed that you could dramatically increase the life span of various animals and organisms by restricting calorie consumption by a large proportion. This has also been validated in humans, where caloric restriction leads to improvements in a range of biomarkers for the aging process. As you could imagine, this is a tough sell for the general public. Most people surveyed usually indicate they would rather live a shorter life than spend the rest of their life eating celery. That includes me.

The other "great hope" of anti-aging supplements – resveratrol, was also found to exert its anti-aging effects via increased autophagy. Resveratrol is the substance extracted from grape skin (or *Japanese knotweed*) which is purported to slow down the aging process. When resveratrol was given to rodents who had their autophagy-related abilities disabled, it failed to give any anti-aging benefits. This appears to indicate that resveratrol perhaps confers some of its benefits via an ability to positively modulate your body's autophagy processes.

Scientists from Sanford-Burnham Medical Research Institute have found a substance that appears to play an important role in autophagy. It is a *transcription factor* (a protein that controls the movement of genetic information from DNA to mRNA) known as *HLH30*. This compound is the first identified transcription factor that is believed to be important in the longevity of *Caenorhabditis elegans* (a type of nematode roundworm) strains. A similar transcription factor, called *TFEB* has been shown to modulated autophagy in mice. Of particular interest is the role that TFEB plays in *Huntington' disease* – possibly the most severe of all genetically-modulated neurodegenerative disorders. Scientists are now studying ways to possibly increase expression of TFEB and reduce the neurotoxicity associated with Huntington's. Again, it appears as if caloric restriction increases expression of TFEB – perhaps pointing to another mechanism driving the anti-aging effect of restricting calories.

Telomere shortening

As mentioned earlier, telomeres sit at the end of chromosomes, gradually shortening after successive replications. Telomeres are often referred to using the rather accurate analogy of the piece of plastic that sits at the end of your shoelaces. Like these plastic caps, telomeres sit at the end of chromosomes, preventing them from "fraying", so to speak. However a more relevant analogy in the case of aging would be a bomb fuse. Telomeres, like a bomb fuse, can shorten to a point before – BOOM! – The cell self-destructs. Sorry, however this bomb analogy is about as exciting as cellular biology gets for some people. If you would permit me a third analogy, the function of telomeres is to act as a kind of fender for the chromosome. The telomere can take all the hits, slowly shortening, while protecting all the valuable DNA stored in the chromosome.

One of the reasons why telomeres shorten as the cell ages is that gradually levels of telomerase decrease. Telomerase adds length to the base of the telomere, slowing down the rate at which it shortens. The activity of telomerase is largely controlled by genes, so in 2010, Harvard researchers investigated the extent to which modulating the telomerase genes could have a beneficial effect on mice. *Jaskelioff et al* indeed found that by reactivating the telomerase activity, they were able to reverse a range of typical biomarkers of aging.

Free-radical theory

By far the most prominent theory on aging is known as the free-radical theory, and states that we gradually accumulate cellular damage caused by free radicals or *reactive oxygen species* (ROS). A free radical is any atom or molecule with an unpaired electron, whereas ROS are a type of free radical specific to oxygen molecules. Free radical damage is typically attributed to superoxide, hydrogen peroxide or peroxynitrite.

Normally electrons exist in pairs and are considered stable. In the case of a free radical with only a single electron, when it meets another molecule it will attempt to steal an electron from that molecule turning it also into a free radical. This can set off a chain reaction which leads to extensive damage at the cellular level through processes such as DNA cross-linking, which have been shown to potentially lead to cancer.

This is where antioxidants come to the rescue. Antioxidants can donate an electron to the free radical molecule without themselves becoming a free radical. Vitamin C is a great example of this, which is why it was the first real mainstream antioxidant that was proposed to counteract the damaging effects of free radicals. More on the use of antioxidants to prevent and reverse free radical damage later.

Unfortunately, ROS have been shown to reliably increase with age. What isn't as clear is which direction the arrow of causation travels. Does aging naturally trigger increased ROS or do elevated ROS accelerate aging? The weight of theoretical and practical evidence points to the latter, however more work is still required.

Mitochondrial dysfunction

The *mitochondrial theory of aging* is actually a sub-set of the *free radical theory*, as the majority of mitochondrial damage is proposed to be caused by free radicals.

Mitochondria are often referred to as your "cellular power plants" as they are responsible for the production of energy at the cellular level. Mitochondria are located in the cytoplasm of each cell (the part of the cell located outside the nucleus but inside the cell wall) and produce the main source of energy for the cell – *adenosine triphosphate* (ATP).

As your mitochondria are so central to the production of the energy which drives many cellular processes, it is unsurprising that scientists have investigated the anti-aging effects of improving mitochondrial function. Indeed, elderly subjects are consistently found to have significant decreases in mitochondrial function compared to younger subject. Two of the supplements with the best research into their positive effects on the mitochondria are coenzyme Q10 (CoQ10 or *ubiquinol*) and D-ribose.

Coenzyme Q10 plays a crucial role in the process of creating ATP at the cellular level, so it is hypothesized that by increasing levels of Co-Q10 by supplementation, you can optimize mitochondrial function to some extent. Co-Q10 is not just at the stage of pure theory or wild speculation. It is now regularly recommended by cardiologists for patients taking statins to reduce cholesterol. Statins reduce the absorption of certain fat soluble nutrients such as vitamin D and Co-Q10 so it is believed that by supplementing with Co-Q10 you are giving some much needed assistance to muscle cells that need Co-Q10 to function properly. This is one of the reasons why statin therapy is often associated with muscle soreness or weakness, as your muscles need these vital fat soluble nutrients for functioning and repair.

One of the reasons why CoQ10 is a no brainer supplement is that is also appears to function as a potent antioxidant. This means that irrespective of whether you believe the *mitochondrial dysfunction* theory or the *free-radical theory*, CoQ10 covers all bases. One of the most notable aspects of oxidative damage by free-radicals is *lipid* (fat) *peroxidation*. This is one of the reasons why CoQ10 is often promoted as a heart healthy supplement – it potently inhibits the oxidation of LDL, the cholesterol transporter molecule implicated in heart disease. CoQ10 reduces this peroxidation by inhibiting the production of *lipid peroxyl radicals*. CoQ10 also recycles other antioxidants such as vitamin E.

Discrepancies in mitochondrial function between males and females may also give us clues as to why women live longer than men on average. Researchers from the Monash School of Biological Sciences and Lancaster University looked at the aging differences between male and female fruit flies *(Side note – if you are wondering why scientists often use fruit flies, it is because they share around 75% of the same genetics as humans and are significantly lower maintenance than rodents and other mammals. If fruit fly research generates positive findings, researchers can move on to mammals and then hopefully on to humans later)*. They found that mitochondrial mutations appear to drive the speed of aging in male fruit flies but to a lesser extent in females. However I should point out that this is confounded by other factors such as the fact that the female immune system appears to retain function later in life compared to males.

Evolutionary theory

Evolution sits at the very heart of this topic as it is the forces of evolution that are largely responsible for our apparently swift descent into mortality. This is largely due to a single, central concept – over countless years, humans have been self-selected for durability against any disease that strikes down someone before they have the opportunity to breed. *Mother Nature* doesn't care if you get cancer or heart disease in your 60s – you have already (in most cases) created progeny to carry your genes. Naturally there are exceptions (including childhood cancers such as leukemia), however in general, if your genetics carry a potential weakness that can strike you down before you reach child-rearing age, as cold and bleak as it sounds, your genetic line will soon die out.

However, if your genetic code holds a predisposition to prostate cancer or heart disease, it will continue to be passed on, as it doesn't impact your ability to pass on your genes.

A version of this idea was one of the very first theories ever proposed to account for the apparent mystery as to why we age. This idea was called *Medawar's Hypothesis* - named after Sir Peter Medawar, famous British zoologist and Nobel Prize winner from the University of London. Nowadays it is usually referred to as the *mutation accumulation theory of aging*. Medawar used the example of *Huntington's disease*, which typically won't strike down someone who carries the genetic predisposition until after they have created offspring. Put another way, over the course of evolution, animals accumulate a range of genetic mutations, however it is only the mutations that cause problems after child rearing age that remain. Any mutations that strike down children or adolescents will soon be weeded out. So, under this theory, aging is simply a range of genetic mutations which have been passed on throughout history.

While this theory is attractive in the sense that it at least hints at the notion that aging is not an inescapable fact of life, there are some problems with it. The most obvious of these is that we now know that gene expression is rather more precise than previously thought when Medawar originally proposed his idea. Genes are typically programmed to express in a particular part of the body and at a particular time in a person's life, so it would be unlikely that animals evolve with the genetic coding to mutate by design during the latter stages of life.

However probably the final nail in the coffin for Medawar's theory was when, as part of the advances in our ability to understand genomics, it was discovered that there are genes for aging and they are not mutations. Some of the genes for aging are closely interwoven with other genes and these genes are often shared by organisms from man all the way to fungi. So clearly spontaneous mutations in one species could not explain the process of aging.

The American evolutionary biologist George Williams, building on the initial work of Medawar, then proposed the *antagonistic pleiotropy hypothesis*, which states that there is an evolutionary cost to every beneficial genetic trait. So when applied to aging it states that we pay the price later in life for everything that has made us a robust species earlier in life. More specifically, it was proposed that aging and senescence was the price we pay for increased fertility and the ability to breed earlier and in greater numbers. However the main problem with this theory as it has not been backed up by the results of any experimentation. If there was an inverse relationship between longevity and fertility, breeding an animal for increased longevity should result in decreased fertility. However, as an example, an experiment using fruit flies found that the specimens bred for longer life actually become more fertile, not less.

To take this concept one step further, many have argued that we are indeed set up like printer cartridges are for *planned obsolescence*. Like a printer cartridge only has so many pages in it before the manufacturer has built in a kind of self-destruct function to boost sales, animals including humans appear to have our own self-destruct built in. This is in the form of various aging processes and diseases that target the elderly. The evolutionary purpose for this is clear – the more a population of animals is burdened by older specimens as a proportion of the total population, the weaker the group is as a whole.

The last of the major evolutionary theories is the *disposable soma theory* (original proposed by the biologist Thomas Kirkwood), which proposes the idea that an organism will prioritize vital functions ahead of repair work, assuming finite resources (finite energy, nutrition etc.). This theory proposes that the number one priority for an organism is to reach reproductive age and this rush to maturity means that other processes such as repair work can be sacrificed. Slowly over time, these small sacrifices accumulate as the aging process.

On the surface this may seem like a plausible theory however there is one major deal-breaker in my opinion – caloric restriction. One of the least disputed ideas in the field of aging is that restricting calories extends the life of an organism. So, under the disposable soma theory, restricting calories should lead to accelerated aging, not decreased aging.

Inflammation and advanced glycation end-products (AGEs)

Inflammation is one of the buzz words in medicine today – and for good reason. Each new emerging study appears to implicate inflammation in a range of diseases from multiple sclerosis to heart disease. Not to mention the conditions which are primarily inflammatory themselves, such as rheumatoid arthritis or inflammatory bowel disease.

Heart disease is the number one killer of middle-aged and older people, so any talk of life extension or anti-aging must take into consideration the mechanisms that underpin heart disease.

A vocal minority of cardiologists have, for some time now, been pointing to the "war on cholesterol" and highlighting something odd. Why in modern times do our arteries appear to suddenly start accumulating cholesterol deposits? If your body is sending cholesterol to your arteries in an attempt to patch up damage, what is causing that damage? Cholesterol is being deposited there for a reason – it's no bad guy. It's just trying to do a job. So the question should be what is causing this damage?

Gradually medical consensus is slowly turning towards chronic arterial inflammation as being a potential culprit. Doctors have known for a long time that heart disease is associated with inflammation – this is why a common test they will often arrange (called a CRP, or *C-reactive protein* test) looks for signs of inflammation. While everyone used to believe that heart disease caused inflammation, now there is a new hypothesis that asks whether inflammation causes heart disease.

Where this gets truly interesting is where there is now a gradually emerging idea that heart disease is not caused by saturated animal fat, but by trans-fatty acids, Omega-6 rich vegetable oils and sugar. Nothing is proven conclusively either way but one powerful piece of evidence is that reducing levels of these three foods in your diet (and keeping saturated fat unchanged or even increased), usually reduces CRP levels.

Put simply, any program that aims to increase longevity must tackle systemic inflammation as a priority. Inflammation damages cells, and each time your body needs to repair damage there is a minute chance of a mutation that could lead to cancer.
Inflammation is one of the factors I can say conclusively is involved in accelerated biological aging.

A recent Yale study published in the journal *Cell Metabolism* identified the *Nlrp3 inflammasome* as the trigger for many of the age-related problems that appear to be either triggered or influenced by inflammation. To put this another way, this study found that the general systemic inflammation which often increases with age isn't a natural consequence, but is turned on by the *Nlrp3 inflammasome*. Where this area of inquiry will get truly interesting is when we are able to prevent *Nlrp3* from doing its job, possibly preventing a range of inflammatory diseases that reduce life expectancy.

Indeed, initial mouse experiments have shown that by reducing the activity of *Nlrp3* the test subjects appeared to be protected from a range of age-related conditions such as dementia, bone loss and glucose intolerance.

Recently Zhang et al, from Albert Einstein College of Medicine found that at least some of the inflammatorily mediated aging we see appears to be related to inflammation in the hypothalamus. The hypothalamus is the part of your brain central to the control of autonomic functions and hormonal control. These researchers found that inflammation in the hypothalamus appeared to trigger a range of age-related health problems such as metabolic syndrome. This inflammation appeared to be controlled by NF-κB (nuclear factor kappa-light-chain-enhancer of activated B cells that regulates transcription of DNA). The researchers found that when they blocked the NF-κB pathway in the hypothalamus, they saw a 20% increase in the longevity of test mice.

Inflammation has also been found to accelerate the production of *advanced glycation end products* (AGEs) which are usually formed when glucose binds with a protein, leading to cellular damage. The most common type of AGE that you would be familiar with is the browning of food, such as when something is caramelized. This is known as the *Maillard reaction* and involves the production of AGEs.

The damaging impact of AGEs in the body appears to be the subject of little debate. As Régis Moreau, Ph.D., a research associate at the Linus Pauling Institute states *"If we can prevent damage or remove existing damage caused by protein glycoxidation and maintain tissue integrity, we may be able to improve the health and vigor of the elderly"*. Stopping the formation of AGEs and repairing the ones that have already formed (or *cross-linked*) is the subject of considerable research at present.

However it should be pointed out that AGEs are not a completely separate aspect of anti-aging research and theory to oxidative stress. AGEs are seen as one of the main triggers for oxidative damage.

A 2010 study published in *Nutrients* also reached the conclusion that *"Although the data are not conclusive, the convergence of data from diverse experimental studies suggests an important role of AGEs in healthy aging, as well as chronic disease morbidity.*
Certainly the data are supportive that endogenous AGEs are associated with declining organ functioning. It appears that dietary AGEs may also be related…As of today, restriction of dietary intake of AGEs and exercise has been shown to safely reduce circulating AGEs, with further reduction in

oxidative stress and inflammatory markers. More research is needed to support these findings and to incorporate these into recommendations for the elderly population."

Interestingly, it is the concerns regarding the formation of AGEs that underpins some of the rationale for the raw food movement, which involves the consumption of uncooked, fresh food. Proponents believe that by avoiding cooked food, they are avoiding the unnecessary addition of AGEs to their diet. This is an interesting theory that deserves more study and it does indeed have logical grounding. However the problem I often observe with both raw food proponents and their vegan equivalents is that they often replace cooked meat with fruit and fruit juice high in fructose – one of the most powerful drivers of oxidative stress caused by AGEs.

Sirtuins

Another exciting field of inquiry at present is a type of protein called a *sirtuin*, which appears to play a role in controlling several aspects of longevity including apoptosis (programmed cell death), inflammation and cellular aging. In fact, if we look in closer detail at why resveratrol is a possible life-extender, it is linked to its ability to activate one of the sirtuins, *SIRT1*.

In a recent issue of *Science*, researchers have found that by targeting the enzyme *SIRT1 deacetylase*, they could achieve spectacular results such as increasing the life-span of rodents by more than 40%. Interestingly, this same pathway (activating SIRT1 deacetylase) appears to be one of the reasons why calorie restriction can work to increase life span.

So while scientists and biotech companies are working hard to develop therapies that specifically target SIRT1, until these new therapies become a reality your only option is resveratrol, caloric restriction or cardiovascular exercise. As if you didn't need another excuse to exercise more. You can now add *"increased SIRT1 deacetylase activity"* to exercise's long list of life-extending benefits. Don't forget to tell your gym buddies this in the locker room. You will be quite the popular one.

There is also considerable excitement regarding *SIRT3*, another sirtuin which is central to the process of mitochondrial function and the generation of stem cells. Researchers from the University of California, Berkeley, found that by up-regulating SIRT3 activity (which usually declines with age), they could reverse some of the markers of aging. Most importantly, increasing SIRT3 activity improves the ability of hematopoietic stem cells to regenerate. The researchers unambiguously said that *"aging-associated degeneration can be reversed by a sirtuin"*.

A commercially available drug that targets either SIRT1 or SIRT3 is a while away, however sirtuin-related therapy appears to be one of the most promising areas of current research into delaying or reversing the aging process. Probably the most likely candidate for being the first "sirtuin activator" available will be NMN (more on this later).

No one has quite "nailed it" yet

Despite the abundance of theories, each with a varying degree of plausibility, no single theory has yet completely nailed down a single reason for exactly why animals age. This is most likely because aging will turn out to be underpinned by a range of different causes.

It is in the area of evolutionary theories in particular, where there are a range of confounding factors that makes it hard to make a convincing case for any single theory. For example, we have the basic theory that aging is helpful for a species as it clears out the weaker, elderly specimens, while preserving the younger generation, making the group as a whole, stronger. However there is an equally convincing case to be made that if we didn't age, we could continue to reproduce ad infinitum. Surely this would lead to greater numbers and therefore a stronger overall group would it not? Or would this just lead to a population explosion (like a rabbit plague, for example) which would deplete resources and lead to the implosion of the group or species? And could you not also say that by allowing the elderly to breed you are increasing the risk of genetic mutations being passed on, if you accept that an organism accumulates transmittable mutations?

Female menopause, on a particular level, appears to give us some indication of how evolution views aging and breeding. On an evolutionary level, menopause appears to exist with the single purpose of preventing an elderly person from reproducing and potentially not being able to care for her young. However this is then confounded by the fact that many species continue to breed for their entire life span.

And if evolution has set up aging as a mechanism to clear out *dead wood* (sorry to sound so clinical), why do so many females live so far past the time where they are fertile? Surely evolution would have set us up like spawning salmon, where we swim upstream to breed and then keel over dead. Salmon are a much better example of evolution only caring about breeding and not life span. But there are too many exceptions for this to be considered a genuine rule of thumb or guiding principle.

Then we have the problem of how different animals age at different rates. If there was a single, underlying factor driving the aging process, surely animals would all age at the same rate. If this was the case, a large dog that was roughly the same weight as a small person would have roughly the same life span. However we know this to not be the case, which is why we have the concept of *dog years*. The maximum life expectancy for a dog is around 15 or 16 years, whereas a human can often reach 80 years. Why do dogs wear out more quickly than humans?

If it was a question of weight, then surely similar animals would age at the same rate due to similar metabolism, heart rate etc. However this argument falls down in far too many examples to be of use. A rat usually lives to 3, while a chipmunk can reach 14. Humans are bigger than smaller animals so perhaps we age more slowly for this reason. However smaller dogs live longer than bigger dogs and humans live almost twice as long as bears. There is not consistent theme here, so I think this is not an area of great potential for us to focus research efforts.

One concept that is a little more consistently applicable is the link between life span and sexual maturity. There does appear to be a link between these two factors. For example, animals that reach sexual maturity more quickly and produce larger numbers o f offspring at a time, tend to have shorter life spans. So, is the relatively long life of a human linked to the time we take to reach sexual maturity and the fact that we only (usually) produce one offspring at a time? Maybe evolution tries to keep animals who breed slowly alive longer so they will have a better chance of creating enough progeny to repopulate. And why exactly do humans take so long to reach sexual maturity? Is it to allow females to grow wide enough hips to give birth to our relatively brain-heavy babies? Or is it because humans lack natural predators, giving us the luxury of taking our time to breed? Scientists have often noted that prey animals breed more quickly than predators, so perhaps they need to rush a little so they are not eaten before they have a chance to reproduce.

It is far too easy to get completely lost in theory here and miss the key point - *Irrespective of why we age, what can we do to increase our chances of reaching 100 and beyond?* That is the focus of the second part of this book.

How to live to 100 and beyond

So now that we are familiar with the various mechanisms that underlie the aging process, we need to apply what we know to increase our potential longevity. However, just tackling the cellular process that drive aging would be far too narrow. What would be the point of taking every anti-aging supplement under the sun if you go ahead and smoke cigarettes or live on junk food?

Therefore, if we are to take a holistic approach to increasing your chances of living to 100, we need to follow a range of general principles so we can tick off each of the factors that encourage a long life and each of the factors that has the chance to strike us down ahead of our time.

Now, let's look at each of these, one by one.

Prevent and reverse oxidative damage

If we are to accept that free radical damage (particularly from reactive oxygen species) is at least part of the cause of the aging process, the next question must be - *how do we stop or reverse this damage?* The answer, as you probably know, is primarily through antioxidants. Think of antioxidants as your fire fighters putting out the fire. However, shouldn't we also endeavor to stop lighting fires? Or, put another way, logically shouldn't we also try to ensure that we do all we can to minimize the creation of free radicals in the first place?

Unfortunately, due to the fact that a large component of free radical generation is unavoidable as a part of oxygen-based metabolism, we are limited in what we can do to minimal the production of them. In fact, after trawling through various research papers and journals, the only credible way I could find to reliably minimize the production of free radicals was to avoid marathon running and minimize UV exposure.

The "marathon running" one usually comes as a shock to people who have been conditioned to view long distance running as a super-healthy activity. Unfortunately this is not the case. Exercise always involves the generation of extra free radicals as a by-product of the ramped-up metabolic processes involved. Usually your body can deal with this extra production of free radicals and this effect is more than offset by the myriad of health benefits you get from cardiovascular exercise. However in the case of regular long distance running, there is such as massive spike in the production of free radicals that your body finds it difficult to keep up in its efforts to neutralize them. This is not new information. For many years now, long distance runners have been instructed to ramp up their consumption of antioxidants such as vitamin C, to help them offset this phenomenon.

Unfortunately for you running buffs out there, the science is turning against long distance running. Various studies have shown that high-intensity interval training (HIIT) tops long distance, steady-state running on just about any metric, from joint wear & tear to fat burning efficiency (i.e. - you can burn more calories in a much shorter period of time).

If running is your passion and it makes you happy (and doesn't ruin your joints), make sure you consume massive amounts of antioxidants through your diet and supplementation.

Anyway, more on this in the Exercise section.

So clearly, our best option for reducing and reversing oxidative damage is via diet and supplementation. But what is the difference between various antioxidants and how do we measure the ability of a substance to neutralize free radicals?

There are so many different antioxidants that I could bore you to death by literally filling an entire book trying to list them all. So instead, I want to focus on the most important and ubiquitous of the antioxidants. But first, let's get a better understanding of how we determine antioxidant capabilities.

How do you determine the antioxidant ability of a particular food?

The globally standardized method for assessing the ability of a substance to scavenge free radicals is a test measuring *oxygen radical absorbance capacity* (ORAC). So a food with a high ORAC score is considered to be high in antioxidant activity.

Whilst the ORAC number gives us a rough guide to antioxidant activity, there is no proven link between an ORAC score and a particular biological benefit. Many scientists believe that the ORAC score of a particular food is meaningless, whereas others believe it still has value as a general guiding principle.

However, if you acknowledge the importance of dietary antioxidants in preventing and reversing oxidative damage, as a general guide, the ORAC score of a particular food is as good as any for informing your understanding. Many people are vehemently opposed to even acknowledging the existence of the ORAC system because of the inherent flaws. They quite rightly point to the fact that there is often little correlation between chemical reactions in a test tube (in-vitro) and what happens in the human body. Also, the ORAC score takes into consideration only one aspect of antioxidant activity. However, my position is that, as long as you consider the ORAC score to be a guide to rough antioxidant activity and not accurate gospel, I have no problems with people trying to include more high ORAC foods into their diets.

Here are the ORAC values for some common[2] foods -

Dark Chocolate 20,823

Pecans 17,940

Walnuts 13,541

Hazelnuts 9,645

Cranberries, raw 9,584

Artichokes 9,416

Kidney beans, red 8,459

Pink beans 8,320

Black beans 8,040

Pistachio nuts 7,983

Currants 7,960

---

[2] Note – I have only focused on commonly available foods. This does not include obscure, hard to find foods.

Pinto beans 7,779

Plums 7,581

Milk chocolate 7,528

Lentils 7,282

Dried apples 6,681

Blueberries 6,552

Prunes 6,552

Soybeans 5,764

Blackberries 5,347

Raw garlic 5,346

Cabernet Sauvignon (red wine variety) 5,034[3]

Raspberries 4,882

Almonds 4,454

Apples, red delicious 4,275

White raisins 4,188

Dates 3,895

Strawberries 3,577

Peanut butter 3,432

Red currants 3,387

Figs 3,383

Cherries 3,365

Gooseberries 3,277

Dried apricots 3,234

Peanuts 3,166

Red cabbage 3,145

Broccoli 3,083

---

[3] I know what you are thinking. Don't even think about it!

Apples 3,082

Raisins 3,037

Pears 2,941

Guava 2,550

Red leaf lettuce 2,380

In terms of pure ORAC punchiness, certain herbs and spices have numbers which dwarf everyday foods. However we tend to use much less quantity, so you need to take that into consideration. However this also shows the importance of eating "real" food. You will never find turmeric or cloves in a Big Mac. Here are some values for spices used commonly in cooking -

Cloves 314,446

Cinnamon 267,536

Oregano 200,129

Turmeric 159,277

Vitamin C

As the most well-known and understood of the antioxidants, vitamin C provides a natural kick-off point for us to look at the different antioxidants. One of the things that primates (including man) have different to other mammals is that we cannot produce vitamin c (ascorbic acid) endogenously - we need to take it in through our diet. Vitamin C is a powerful scavenger of free radicals such as hydrogen peroxide, one of the most potentially damaging free radicals.

Fortunately a healthy diet rich in fruits and vegetables is likely to have good levels of vitamin c. A clinical vitamin c deficiency (scurvy, which, in times past would afflict sailors who did not have ready access to fresh food) is therefore relatively rare in the western world. However there is a massive gap between the minimum amount needed to avoid scurvy and the amount needed to prevent oxidative damage.

As well as treating oxidative stress, vitamin C is vital for a range of important reactions in the body and brain, such as the production on certain neurotransmitters and hormones.

In general I prefer to get vitamin c from food rather than supplements, however I am a fruit fanatic so this is not hard for me. If, for whatever reason, you can't get your vitamin C from food, then supplementation is the next best thing.

I would aim for a minimum of 500mg each day, in divided doses because vitamin C, being water soluble, cannot be stored in the body. Some of the foods highest in vitamin C include - peppers (capsicum), citrus fruit, kiwi fruit, guava, leafy green vegetables and berries.

In general, vitamin C is perfectly safe, with a couple of exceptions applying to supplements only. If vitamin C gives you gastrointestinal distress, stick to buffered types of vitamin C such as *calcium ascorbate*. Also, if you have been diagnosed with cancer and are currently undergoing treatment, only take vitamin C (or any other supplement at all) with your doctor's permission. There are certain scenarios where taking antioxidants during cancer treatment can have a paradoxically pro-oxidant effect.

Vitamin E

Vitamin E is actually a single term for a collection of various fat-soluble compounds that protect cells from free radical damage. Vitamin E is important in a different way to the water-soluble vitamin C, as it also targets the free radicals that are produced as a by-product of fat oxidation. As we heard earlier, oxidized LDL is one of the most damaging types of free radicals. The other piece of good news is that vitamin E and vitamin C act synergistically, both playing a role (a kind of "one-two punch" act) in neutralizing the same free radical molecule.

As with vitamin C, the benefits of vitamin E for conferring longevity benefits are not limited to free radical scavenging. Vitamin E has long been promoted as a "heart-healthy" supplement because it makes your arterial walls less sticky and inhibits platelet aggregation, both implicated in heart disease.

In general, as vital as vitamin E is, the evidence for its use as a supplement is not yet compelling enough. Or, put another way, a little bit of vitamin E in the diet is great, with more not necessarily better.

My favorite sources for vitamin E are nuts and avocado, both "super-foods" in their own right. Remember though – peanuts are not nuts (although they are indeed high in Vitamin E).

Astaxanthin

As if you didn't need another reason to take krill oil.

Krill oil contains a super-potent carotenoid antioxidant called *astaxanthin*, which appears to have significantly greater free radical scavenging activity than vitamin C and vitamin E. This appears to be linked to its ability to donate electrons (and thereby neutralizing free radicals) and continue to function, due to its surplus of electrons. As you will remember from earlier, typically an antioxidant will be broken down and recycled once it has done its job of donating an electron to a free radical. Most antioxidant molecules can also only deal with one free radical molecule at a time, whereas astaxanthin can neutralize a large number of free radicals simultaneously by surrounding them in an *electron cloud*. When I first read about how astaxanthin functions, I imagined that it must look like a kind of "antioxidant terminator" as it annihilates any free radical in its path.

Astaxanthin has recently been the subject of increasing interest and excitement from medical researchers due to the wide range of potential benefits it confers, such as reducing inflammation and preventing free radical damage in the eyes.

However its ability to protect the brain and cardiovascular system is where the bulk of recent research has been focused. It appears to have a particularly prominent ability to fight cognitive decline in the elderly by neutralizing phospholipid hydroperoxides, one of the hypothesized causes of Alzheimer's disease. In terms of cardiovascular effects, it appears to lower blood pressure, decrease triglycerides and increase HDL levels.

Another massive benefit over other carotenoids (such as beta carotene), is that in high doses, astaxanthin retains its antioxidant effects. Other carotenoids can become pro-oxidant in high doses. One of the reasons why it is not recommended to ever supplement with vitamin A or beta-carotene.

A good indicator of the usefulness of a particular substance is how often I mention it in different contexts. Astaxanthin is a name you will hear repeatedly in this book. Not only does it do all the above mentioned beneficial things in your body, a study even found that it reduced c-reactive protein (CRP), the key biomarker of inflammation, by more than 20%, without the inherent dangers associated with anti-inflammatory drugs. Inflammation is a topic I cover multiple times, as it is implicated in everything from heart disease, to depression, to premature cellular aging.

The best sources of astaxanthin are krill oil supplements and wild-caught salmon. Astaxanthin is what gives each of these their pinkish-red color. This bears repeating - krill oil should be a compulsory addition to your anti-aging arsenal. It is as close as we get to a miracle pill.

I am currently writing a standalone guide to astaxanthin which I hope to release soon, so check my Amazon author page in late May 2015, unless I get side-tracked in the meantime!

Polyphenols and Flavonoids

I am not particularly enamored with reductionist thinking, as it tends to be overly simplistic. Like when you are told that depression is "caused by low serotonin" or that a particular food is healthy simply because it is high in vitamin C.

Likewise, any attempts to isolate the anti-aging benefits of various fruits and vegetables down to a single vitamin or mineral would be misguided.

The perfect example of this is when we look at the various polyphenols and flavonoids that certain fruit and vegetables contain. Simply isolating one of these particular substances and putting it into a pill rarely demonstrates the same health effects as just eating a piece of fruit.

Flavonoids (which are a type of polyphenol, or polyphenolic compound) have been the subject of considerable excitement in recent years. Have you noticed all those reports detailing the health benefits of green tea, blueberries and red wine? These are largely related to the various flavonoids that each of these foods (and drinks) contains.

One of the reasons why I feel the focus on single vitamins in food is misguided is that each day (assuming you eat a healthy diet) your consumption of various flavonoids far outweighs your consumption of, for example, vitamin C. Flavonoids are one of the reasons why you should be excited about fruits and vegetables and maximize your consumption of them.

One of the beauties of flavonoids is that they can target different aspects of oxidative stress concurrently. Depending on which particular flavonoid we are talking about, they can target not only oxidized LDL but also reactive oxygen species such as hydrogen peroxide as well.

Flavonoids are potent antioxidants that you should endeavor to make part of your daily diet. Don't worry about popping any particular pill. If you have a diet rich in multi-colored fruits and vegetables you should have most of your bases covered. The reason for the multi-colored requirement is that various flavonoids and polyphenols have different colors, so if you included a wide range of colors in your diet, you are almost certainly getting broad-spectrum antioxidant coverage.

However there are certain foods and drinks that have a particularly potent concentration of powerful flavonoids. You should try to include the following into your diet where possible -

Tea

A perfect example of the reason why it is difficult to be reductionist about the health effects of certain foods is good old fashioned tea (*camellia Sinensis*). Not only does tea contain potent antioxidants known as *catechins*, it also contains L-theanine, an amino acid that has relaxation-inducing and mood-brightening effects.

The main catechin found in tea is called *epigallocatechin gallate* (EGCG) and is found mostly in green tea and white tea (black tea loses a lot of the catechin activity due to the extra processing step needed). EGCG has been found in various animal and laboratory studies to inhibit the development of certain cancers. However it should be pointed out that this was under mega-dosing conditions - far in excess of the levels you would get from drinking tea. Some companies are now working on developing concentrated forms of EGCG as a potential cancer preventative or treatment.

However, in the meantime, the ability of EGCG to work as an antioxidant is not disputed.

Tea would be considered a "super-food" simply based on its catechin content, however the good news doesn't stop there. Green tea is also a potent *thermogenic* (it increases metabolic rate, leading to potential fat loss). If we accept that overweight and obesity are a major driver of premature mortality, this must also be considered as a factor in evaluating tea's longevity-promoting effects.

Another bonus is the L-theanine content I just mentioned. L-theanine has been shown to increase levels of dopamine and to a lesser extent, serotonin, in the brain. Unsurprisingly, L-theanine is now a popular supplement for those needing a mood-boost or sleep improvement.

More on theanine and EGCG in the section on nootropics.

Berries

One of the main reasons why you would have seen blueberries plastered around everywhere as a "super-food" is because they contain a potent flavonoid known as *anthocyanin*. This flavonoid, which gives berries their dark red and purple color, has been shown to potently inhibit the oxidation of fats. A study published in the *Journal of Biomedicine and Biotechnology* found that anthocyanin had a beneficial effect on the cardiovascular system by preventing lipid oxidation. Another study conducted by the U.S. Department of Agriculture's Human Nutrition Research Center on Aging at Tufts University, found that anthocyanin ameliorated age-related losses of cognitive function in rodents.

Another reason to include liberal amounts of berries in your diet is that they are relatively low in fructose. Despite what you may have read, fruit should not be consumed in unlimited amounts. At a certain point, the antioxidant benefits will be outweighed by the damaging effects of fructose. This can be mitigated to a certain extent by focusing on low-fructose fruits such as berries.

Resveratrol

One exception to my usual rule of focusing on real foods as your main source of antioxidants is resveratrol. This is because the most common source of resveratrol that people focus on is red wine. Anything up to a third of a glass of red wine per day is net-positive for your health, however if you go beyond this, the negative effects of alcohol will outweigh the benefits of the extra resveratrol.

Over the past few years, resveratrol has become the darling of the life-extension community due to some interesting research results. Studies have shown the ability to lengthen telomeres, reduce blood sugar, reduce inflammation and even extend the life of certain basic organisms such as fruit flies and worms. Similarly, a study on fish showed a significant life-span enhancing effect (more than 50%) with resveratrol.

Various cancer-related studies have also shown that, in certain situations, resveratrol has the ability to either prevent cancer or reduce the size of existing cancers. This is all preliminary research however, so please do not view resveratrol as a proven cancer-fighter just yet until more research is available.

In the brain, resveratrol has also been shown to reduce the formation of *beta-amyloid plaque*, which is thought to be the main cause of Alzheimer's disease. Again, this is all preliminary stuff, although interesting and promising nonetheless.

In terms of the alcohol issue, the way I look at it is - if you are determined to drink alcohol, at least stick to red wine to get the modest cardio-protective and resveratrol-related benefits. However please do not fool yourself by thinking you are extending your life-span by chugging cheap pinot noir every night.

A much better option is to take a resveratrol supplement. These usually contain resveratrol from the world's richest known source - *Japanese knotweed*.

However, as mentioned in the introduction, my recommendations regarding resveratrol come with rather sizable caveats. Most likely due to poor bioavailability, resveratrol has recently been a poor performer in clinical trials, with serum tests showing very little actual resveratrol present after oral consumption. However the good news is that researchers are hard at work developing more bioavailable forms.

In the meantime, unless you have unlimited money to spend on consuming large quantities, I withhold any strong support for taking it as a supplement.

Glutathione – The "master antioxidant"

Inside your body there is a simple molecule which you have possibly never heard of, yet is integral to both your physical health and the speed at which you age. This molecule is *glutathione*. It is so important that it is sometimes referred to as the *master antioxidant* or the *mother of all antioxidants*. This is not just hyperbole either. I will get to why in a moment.

Due to the fact that glutathione contains organically bonded sulfur (via the amino acids that make up glutathione), glutathione is the most powerful single way to reduce oxidative stress and detoxify. Sulfur is a sticky molecule that binds to reactive oxygen species and certain toxins, rendering them inactive.

Often in natural health books or websites, you will read the term "detoxify" in vague, nebulous ways. You will hear that sweating helps you detoxify (it doesn't – you don't eliminate toxins via the skin) or that you need to go on a "detox diet". Rarely will you even be told what these nefarious "toxins" are.

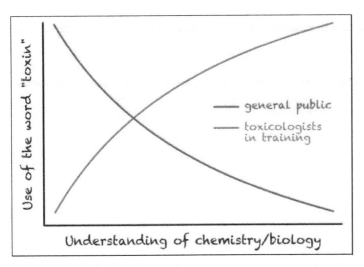

Source - Unknown

However, as I pointed out in my guides on milk thistle and liver detoxification supplements, there are occasions where the term "detoxify" is apt. Typically these occasions refer to increasing the ability of your liver to detoxify various substances (such as acetaminophen, which I will get to in a moment) and by increasing levels of glutathione.

The most powerful example of why glutathione is so important is the case of acetaminophen (paracetamol in certain countries) overdose. If you or one of your pets takes a massive dose of acetaminophen, left untreated it will often lead to liver failure and then death. The reason for this is that your liver uses glutathione to neutralize acetaminophen, which is a harmful toxin for your body. After receiving a massive dose of acetaminophen, you literally run out of glutathione, leading to the accumulation of acetaminophen in your liver. At a certain point your liver then shuts down.

This is how important glutathione is.

However where this gets truly interesting is when we look at one of the treatments for acetaminophen overdose. This substance also happens to be my number one supplement for optimizing glutathione levels - *N-acetylcysteine*. Yes, the same substance given intravenously to overdose patients is also available as an over the counter (OTC) supplement.

Importantly, glutathione is not just vital as an antioxidant in its own right, it also functions to boost the effectiveness of other antioxidants such as vitamin C, vitamin E and lipoic acid.

As glutathione levels gradually decrease as you age, it has been suggested as one of the central players in the aging process and certain diseases associated with age.

Unfortunately you can't just take glutathione as a pill, so the only way to increase levels is to take in the precursors of glutathione via your diet or supplementation. The easiest way to boost levels via your diet is to consume foods rich in precursor amino acids such as cysteine (which contains sulfur). The best foods for this are cruciferous vegetables such as broccoli, along with sulfur-rich foods such as garlic or onions.

However the most powerful single way to increase levels of glutathione is by supplementation. Here are my picks for supplements that boost glutathione levels -

N-acetylcysteine (NAC)

As I mentioned earlier, NAC has a long history of use in medicine - particularly for the treatment of acute paracetamol (acetaminophen) overdose and for breaking up the thick mucus associated with conditions such as cystic fibrosis.

In recent years, due to the wide range of beneficial effects that NAC has on the body, it has become increasingly popular as a supplement. All too often, the latest 'buzz' supplement turns out to be mostly hot air. However, NAC is one substance where I can vouch for its powerful and positive effects on the liver and brain. Interestingly, NAC is also one supplement where both the 'natural health' people and the medical community are in agreement. I was reminded of this the other day when a friend visited a specialist for fibromyalgia. As well as several different pain and sleep medications, the specialist had also recommended a daily dose of NAC. It is not often you leave a specialist's office with a recommendation to take supplements!

What is NAC?

NAC is closely related to the amino acid cysteine, with a few minor chemical differences. This does not really tell us much about it at all, so it is best to discuss what it does rather than what it is. And the best way to look at that is to refer back to why NAC is used for paracetamol overdose.

As I previously mentioned, an overdose of paracetamol depletes the liver of glutathione which is needed to clear the toxic levels of the drug from your body. This kind of overdose is the most common cause of acute liver failure in the US today. NAC is one of the most potent agents available for increasing glutathione.

Remember, NAC has the support of both the alternative medicine and the scientific community. According to Stanford University's Dr. Kondala R. Atkuri, *"NAC has been used successfully to treat glutathione deficiency in a wide range of infections, genetic defects and metabolic disorders, including HIV infection and Chronic Obstructive Pulmonary Disease. Over two-thirds of 46 placebo-controlled clinical trials with orally administered NAC have indicated beneficial effects of NAC measured either as trial endpoints or as general measures of improvement in quality of life and well-being of the patients."*

For example, a trial with results published in the November 2006 journal *Apoptosis*, looked at whether NAC could stop or reverse liver cell death in subjects with life-threatening liver failure. Based on results with animal test subjects, researchers reached the conclusion that NAC showed a clear liver-protective benefit in this situation. Another study which was published in the January 2008 edition of the journal *Liver Transplantation*, found that children who received NAC for acute liver failure had a better survival rates and positive health outcomes than those not receiving NAC.

Apart from its use in emergency wards to prevent liver failure, NAC is also used for a wide range of other illnesses and diseases –

* NAC has been shown to protect against some strains of influenza

* NAC is sometimes used to treat chronic obstructive pulmonary disease (COPD)

* NAC has been shown reduce oxidative stress caused by exercise (note - this doesn't mean that exercise is bad for you - it means that intense or long duration exercise can increase some types of harmful oxidative stress)

* NAC improves insulin sensitivity in patients with type 2 diabetes or other forms of insulin resistance and metabolic derangement.

* NAC has been shown to improve both schizophrenia and bipolar disorder. However at this stage, the mechanism of action remains unclear. It is believed that one of the main reasons is that NAC modulates NMDA receptors and the overall level of glutamate in the brain. However this is not yet proven and there could be another mechanism of action at work.

* NAC has been used to treat marijuana and cocaine addiction with success

* NAC is often used on HIV patients due to its immune-stimulating effects

* NAC can be used to chelate (detoxify) the body of heavy metals such as mercury and also prevent damage to internal organs such as the kidneys, by mercury and other heavy metals.

* NAC has also been trialed as a treatment for *Sjogren's syndrome*. NAC was shown to reduce eye pain in a recent study.

 * NAC has also been shown to act as a potent anti-inflammatory due to the reduction of oxidative stress (due to its antioxidant action) and also its ability to reduce levels of pro-inflammatory substances in the body such as *IL-6 (interleukin 6)*. Remember, widespread inflammation puts additional stress on the liver.

* Due to both its antioxidant and anti-inflammatory actions, along with other mechanisms of action such as preventing DNA damage, NAC has been shown to inhibit the development of various cancers.

* NAC has been shown to increase release of the neurotransmitter dopamine and protect against the damage of dopamine receptors in the brain from chronic amphetamine use.

* NAC has been shown to dramatically decrease levels of *lipoprotein (a)*. A recent trial showed that oral NAC decreased levels of lipoprotein (a) by 70%. High levels of Lipoprotein (a) have been associated with increased risk of heart disease, so by bringing down levels of lipoprotein (a) NAC has shown some promise in this area.

Alpha lipoic acid – The fat & water-soluble powerhouse

Alpha lipoic acid (ALA) is a compound produced in the body which acts as a co-factor for the production of vital energy from the metabolism of branched-chain amino acids. This energy production occurs at the cellular level – in our mitochondria, which we were familiar with from earlier in the book. In this respect, ALA works at the same level as another very important co-factor - co-enzyme Q10 (*Co-Q10* or *ubiquinone*). Think back to science class and how chemical reactions require different agents. In your body, substances such as ALA and Co-Q10 are necessary for certain energy-producing reactions.

ALA acts as an antioxidant by scavenging various reactive oxygen species (ROS) and is one of the only antioxidants that is both water and fat soluble. Antioxidants are typically either one or the other and therefore have a mode of action in specific parts of the body. For example, Vitamin C is water soluble but not fat soluble, whereas Vitamin E and Vitamin A are fat soluble, not water soluble. Often the best way to tell is by the tablet they come in. Vitamin E and A usually come in transparent gel caps (like fish oil tables), whereas Vitamin C is usually a powder or tablet made from powder. ALA is not just water and fat soluble - it also recycles other antioxidants and similar substances such as Vitamin E, Co-Q10 and glutathione.

ALA's ability to scavenge free radicals has been backed up by extensive testing which has shown that ALA decreases urinary *isoprostanes*, *oxidized LDL* and *plasma protein carbonyls*, which are biomarkers of oxidative stress in the body. I should also point out that oxidized LDL is one of the strongest known factors in the potential development of heart disease via inflammation of the arteries.

Also, it is important to note that, like N-acetylcysteine, ALA is not just a substance limited to the world of alternative health. In countries such as Germany, ALA is a recognized gold-standard treatment for various neuropathies (nerve pain disorders) such as diabetic neuropathy, due primarily to its ability to increase aortic blood flow. This bears emphasizing - ALA is a substance with documented, identifiable and beneficial effects on the human body.

Despite the range of beneficial effects that ALA has on the body, it is the ability of ALA to recycle and increase levels of glutathione that for me is of most interest in the context of anti-aging.

Despite the body of evidence, ALA as a means to increase levels of glutathione is taking longer to catch on than more well-known substances such as NAC or milk thistle. And this is not due to a lack of studies - in fact the first major human trial was conducted way back in the 1970s by the National Institutes of Health (NIH). The results of even this very first trial were amazing - out of 79 people with severe liver damage, 75 recovered full liver function after a period using ALA. As recently as 1999, there was a follow up trial by the same researchers using a combination of ALA, silymarin (milk thistle) and selenium in patients with liver disease. All patients recovered liver function and did not require subsequent transplants - a remarkable result when you consider how little-known this substance is. The mechanism by which this was achieved was through the glutathione boosting effect.

Selenium

Selenium is a trace element that plays an important function assisting glutathione in neutralizing free radicals such as hydrogen peroxide. More specifically, selenium is a co-factor in the production of glutathione peroxidase, which targets and neutralizes reactive oxygen species such as hydrogen peroxide.

Selenium is another classic example of "little is good, too much is very bad", as it is toxic in high doses. Selenium is not something I recommend you supplement with. If you eat a healthy diet with a wide range of different foods, you are unlikely to be deficient.

There have been a range of studies that implicate selenium deficiency in a wide range of conditions such as cancer and diabetes, however actual trials have failed to show any benefit for selenium supplementation.

However, others believe that selenium deficiency is more common than is currently reported. Renowned author of *"The Four-Hour Body"*, Tim Ferriss, is one example of someone who discovered that they had a selenium deficiency. In Ferriss' case, it manifested in the form of low testosterone, so, when he fixed his selenium deficiency, his testosterone status normalized.

If you suspect a selenium deficiency, you can easily get it tested. Just request this test with your doctor. However a much easier option is to religiously eat two Brazil nuts every day. That should give you just the right amount of selenium for optimal functioning.

Do I need to take supplements?

In terms of your own requirements for supplementation, you should be guided by -

- Your probable level of oxidative stress and toxin insult. If you consume a lot of alcohol and junk food, smoke, or are in environments with high levels of toxins (such as China and the airborne mercury issue), you will need more.

- Your consumption of sulfur rich foods such as cruciferous vegetables, onions and garlic. If you eat a diet high in sulfur rich foods, you may need less supplementation support.

- Your genetics. Some people have impaired function of the GSTM1 gene, which is required for normal glutathione activity. These people need to supplement to provide additional support to their glutathione synthesis pathway.

Healthy weight

How many obese 80 year olds do you see? If you think back to all the centenarians you have seen on television being celebrated for reaching this important milestone, what was their typical body type? All pretty thin weren't they?

Not only does being overweight dramatically increase your chance of dying by cardiovascular disease and certain types of cancers, it triggers a range of biological changes that age you more quickly than those at a healthy weight. Not only does being overweight expose you directly to increased mortality, it causes primary illnesses that can then lead to early death or accelerated aging. Type 2 diabetes is a classic example of this. At a cellular level, getting type 2 diabetes is like stepping into an aging acceleration machine.

Recently, scientists have identified clear links between body fat percentage and cellular aging. For example a recent study which looked at more than a thousand women of various ages found that as the body weight increased, telomere length shortened. This is believed to be driven by levels of the hunger/satiety hormone *leptin* which is stored in fat cells. The higher the level of leptin, the shorter the telomere. As an aside, the same study also found that smokers have shorter telomeres than non-smokers. But that's not particularly surprising right? Nothing surprising there. What is more surprising is that being overweight was associated with shorter telomeres than smoking was! Now that I found surprising.

A study published in 2009 in the journal Nature, found that *"Obesity accelerates the aging of adipose tissue, a process only now beginning to come to light at the molecular level. Experiments in mice suggest that obesity increases the formation of reactive oxygen species in fat cells, shortens telomeres—and ultimately results in activation of the p53 tumor suppressor, inflammation and the promotion of insulin resistance."*

No one wants to reach 100 and have no quality of life, and one of the biggest factors in quality of life is mobility. Lacking mobility dramatically reduces the activities you can enjoy as you get older. Not to mention the fact that extended periods sitting down is associated with lower life expectancy. Also key is the disturbing tendency of people to suddenly go downhill and die soon after breaking a hip in old age.

Being overweight is extremely taxing on your skeletal system and increases your chances of suffering from various forms of osteoarthritis. This is compounded by the fact that being overweight itself, reduces your ability to engage in the kinds of healthy exercise that helps protect against arthritis later in life.

However it is important to note that more isn't always better. If there is on consistent point I like to make is that you should always look for balance. If we look at the other end of the spectrum from overweight people, we will find ex-athletes. It is one of the great tragedies of competitive sport that when athletes retire, they are often struck down from various injuries that have come from a life of over-use. Particularly bad is the arthritis that often sets in where there has been a previous injury sustained - such as that seen in knee ligaments.

So where possible, if you plan on leading a long life of optimal mobility, your focus needs to be on low-impact exercises. One of the most hotly debated topics in physical fitness at the moment is the recent understanding that long-distance running is actually net-negative due to both the spectacularly high level of oxidative stress and the negative effects on the joints of many years of long-distance running. Previously, marathon running was held up as a paragon of healthy living, until healthy professionals started pointing out that they were seeing a lot of long-distance runners with knees and ankles completely shot.

Fortunately, we now know that you can achieve the positive health benefits of exercise with much less strain on your joints by either engaging in low impact exercise or focusing on high intensity interval training (HIIT - as mentioned in the section on exercise). Researchers have found that the same weight loss benefits can be achieved with short periods of intense exercise, compared to long periods pounding the pavement at a medium intensity (this type of exercise is called steady-state exercise as the intensity stays roughly consistent during each session). The way they measure this is by putting them on a bike and measuring their *VO2 max* (also known as *maximal aerobic capacity*), which is a fairly reliable measure of energy expenditure.

Therefore, to ensure that you get the benefits of exercise without putting undue wear and tear on your musculoskeletal system, the following types of exercise could be a good starting point. Note that I have included yoga below. Unless doing intense forms of *Ashtanga* yoga or some of the more advanced *Iyengar* series of poses, yoga is generally not a particularly effective form of cardiovascular work. However, what it does have going for it, is the unrivalled ability to improve mobility. You can see this when you see elderly yoga adepts, who move like someone significantly younger than they are. However in the interests of balance I should also mention a counterpoint to the argument that yoga prevents injury. Some experts in physiology believe that yoga can also be harmful as it increases range of motion to such as degree that there is an increased risk of hyper-extension related injuries. Even if this was correct, I think it applies to a small subset of the population who are doing very heavy lifting in the weights room.

Here are some potential options for suitable forms of exercise -

- Swimming

- Yoga

- Pilates

- Cycling

- Ping-Pong (also excellent for building hand-eye co-ordination)

- Weight training (it's no use being in shape if you have no muscles supporting your skeletal system)

- Walking

- Rowing

- Rollerblading (chance of injury however)

- Water aerobics

Before I go, I need to point out one more thing. Being underweight is also not healthy. Sorry to bang on about it however the key is balance. When you are dramatically underweight, your body assumes that you are in a famine and undergoes a variety of processes. The most obvious of which is that in dangerously thin women, their menstruation stops. And this is not just limited to the painfully thin. New research suggests that someone with excellent muscle definition due to low body-fat percentage is also not the ideal. Your body needs some body fat as an energy buffer and for various biological processes. A little bit of body fat is good, too much is very, very bad.

Reduce inflammation

In terms of supplements that reduce levels inflammation in the body, there are two which I consider virtually compulsory - omega 3 fatty acids and curcumin. While both are potent anti-inflammatories, they operate via different pathways, with a range of consequent benefits throughout the body. Based on the latest research I am reading, I would now also as astaxanthin to this list, considering how beneficial it is for a variety of reasons and not just inflammation.

Omega 3 Fatty Acids

Like several other important nutrients and supplements, a testament to the body-wide benefits of omega 3 is the fact that I could have included it in a number of sections, from the brain to the cardiovascular system. However I believe that it is one particular mechanism that drives the majority of all the omega 3-related benefits - its ability to switch the body from a *pro*-inflammatory to an *anti*-inflammatory state. To learn why it does this, we will need to also look at omega 6 fatty acids and the sometimes yin-yang relationship between these two vital fats.

Omega 3, in the form of fish oil or krill oil tablets, along with the consumption of healthy seafood, is one of the most important things you can do for your brain and body in terms of increasing longevity.

If we first look to the brain, one of the key factors that enables the quick and efficient transfer of information around your brain is the health of your myelin, which is a fatty sheath that covers your nerves. And yes, you guessed it, your myelin is essentially made of omega 3. You may have heard what happens when your myelin become damaged and dysfunctional - multiple sclerosis (MS), which is a debilitating, progressive neurological disorder. We do not yet know the cause of multiple sclerosis, however inflammation (and potentially vitamin D deficiency) is strongly implicated.

However it is omega 3's role as a potent anti-inflammatory that underlies most of the beneficial effects we see with this amazing fatty acid. In your brain and body, we can say (for illustration purposes) that inflammation is controlled by omega 6 (which increases inflammation) and Omega 3 (which decreases it). Remember, inflammation is not dangerous in itself - without inflammation your body would not be able to heal certain injuries and fight illness. The problems only emerge when the balance between omega 3 and omega 6 gets of out of whack. The theory as to why inflammation today runs rampant in humans is that in the past, our diets were more skewed to omega 3 rich foods. However today, with our grain-based diet, we consume far too much omega 6 and not enough omega 3. Not only do we consume a large amount of grain, our animals are now also mainly fed grains and oilseeds (corn, wheat, barley, soybean meal) instead of grass, so our meat is also now high in Omega 6.

The single best thing you can do to rectify this is to take a large dose of fish oil or krill oil.

Certain research suggests that krill may be better absorbed and it also contains astaxanthin, so if your budget can stretch, I highly recommend krill supplements.

There is a fascinating area of research recently which hypothesizes that depression may be associated with elevated levels of inflammation in the brain. As this is early days, scientists don't yet know whether inflammation causes depression or whether depression causes inflammation, however it is certainly a promising line of inquiry. Due to the fact that many sufferers of depression have indicated that omega 3 appears to help them, this would make perfect sense.

My preference is to get your omega 3 from a wide-range of sources. Omega 3 contains two important substances - DHA (*docosahexaenoic acid*) and EPA (*eicosapentaenoic acid*). Each source of omega 3 has different ratios of these two substances and different levels of absorption by your body. The most common sources of omega 3 include - fish oil, krill oil, cod liver oil* (which also contains vitamin D and vitamin A), seafood** (particularly fatty fish), grass-fed beef and eggs.

Due to the fact that cod liver oil also contains Vitamin A, you should be careful to keep your consumption of this at reasonable levels. In some instances, high levels of Vitamin A can be toxic for humans. More is not always better.

** *Be careful to keep your consumption of certain fish that are high in mercury to sensible levels. In general, fish at the top of the food chain such as sharks, tuna or swordfish, are the main offenders you need to be careful of.*

Curcumin

One of the most exciting developments to come out of scientific research in recent years has been the growing understanding of the benefits of curcumin for the human body. Curcumin, which is extracted from turmeric (yes, the same turmeric used in Indian curries), has a long history in certain cultures for treating a range of complaints. The good news is that these traditional claims are now being backed up by rigorous, placebo-controlled clinical trials.

The range of effects that curcumin has on the body is surprisingly extensive, however most attention has been given to curcumin's abilities as an anti-inflammatory, anti-depressant and anti-cancer agent.

Firstly, what exactly is curcumin, and the turmeric plant from which it is extracted?

Turmeric, or curcuma longa, is a member of the ginger family. It is a perennial plant which grows to about 5-6 feet tall in the tropical regions of southern Asia. Turmeric has been used for over 4000 years both as a medicinal herb as well as a spice for cooking. It is fragrant, with a bitter and sharp character to taste.

It is made up of three main compounds; *desmethoxycurcumin, bis-desmethoxycurcumin* and *curcumin*, with curcumin being the most active *curcuminoid* of the turmeric plant and hence where the majority of attention is focused. In traditional medicine and naturopathic modalities, such as India's Ayurvedic system, turmeric has been used to treat a wide range of problems including arthritis, jaundice, heartburn (dyspepsia), stomach pain, diarrhea, intestinal gas, stomach bloating, appetite loss, liver issues, gallbladder disorders, laryngitis, bronchitis, diabetes, headaches, bronchitis, lung infections, fibromyalgia, colds, leprosy and cancer. Now, that is a pretty long list and naturally many of these traditional applications have not yet been verified by enough scientific evidence to be recommended by the medical community. There are quite a few studies already underway, looking to determine if curcumin demonstrates any ability to manage or treat arthritis, stomach ulcers, Alzheimer's disease and high cholesterol.

However, that doesn't mean that curcumin hasn't already been extensively studied. In PubMed (the database of various clinical trials), curcumin is cited almost 4000 times, with strong evidence to suggest effectiveness – as an antioxidant, anti-inflammatory, anti-atherosclerotic, preventing liver and kidney toxicity, as a potential treatment for psoriasis, diabetes, multiple sclerosis, Alzheimer's, HIV disease, septic shock, cardiovascular disease, lung fibrosis, arthritis, and inflammatory bowel disease!

That long list alone would be sufficient to justify further studies, however curcumin also shows in vitro (i.e. – in a test tube essentially, not in a human or animal subject) anti-cancer benefits, appearing to treat a number of cancers including breast, colon, kidney, liver, basal cell carcinoma, prostate, melanoma and also leukemia.

The single greatest negative health consequence of the modern-day inflammation epidemic is the incidence of heart disease. Many people do not realize that inflammation of the cardiovascular system is behind the majority of incidences of heart disease. For a long time, cholesterol has been the 'bad guy' – and unfairly so. Blaming cholesterol for heart disease is like blaming a fireman for a fire. The cholesterol is just there to put out the fire (inflammation).

However irrespective of what is causing inflamed arteries, curcumin is proving to be a potent treatment for arterial inflammation alongside other substances such as Omega 3 fatty acids. Various studies have shown that curcumin is able to suppress or reverse the effects of certain pro-inflammatory substances in the body such as *cytokines*.

Curcumin's benefit for the liver appears to be only slightly related to its potent anti-inflammatory properties. In terms of the liver, it is the fact that curcumin is a potent antioxidant and booster of glutathione levels which is behind the liver-healing effects of this amazing substance.

Clinical studies have shown that curcumin possesses the rare ability to massively boost your body's ability to produce glutathione and keep your liver in perfect condition (along with N-acetylcysteine, alpha lipoic acid and milk thistle). For example, researchers at the Medical University Graz in Austria revealed that curcumin as a compound delays the onset of liver damage caused by cirrhosis.

Curcumin has also been shown to boost the production of bile, assisting the liver in its efforts to digest dietary fat. The evidence has been sufficiently strong for the German Commission E (the scientific advisory board for Germany's equivalent of the Food & Drug Administration) to approves turmeric as a treatment for gastrointestinal problems.

Curcumin has stood up to a massive amount of testing to confirm its safety. Amazingly, it has been associated with no obvious toxic effects on the body. On the contrary, several studies have shown that administration of curcumin reduces the toxicity of other poisons such as arsenic.

If I was forced to imagine a potential downside, it could be in cases where some degree of inflammation is required and curcumin suppresses this. However, this scenario would be exceedingly rare. The human inflammation system is an 'over-reacting' system. This means that it usually creates inflammation far in excess of what is required, as, in evolutionary terms, this would be the better outcome for the body. As curcumin only reduces inflammation and doesn't eliminate it altogether, I would still think that there would be very few occasions where curcumin could be dangerous due to its anti-inflammatory properties.

As curcumin reduces clotting, it would be advisable to avoid curcumin leading up to any surgery, as the body's clotting ability is vital after any major procedure. Curcumin should not be taken along with blood thinners such as Warfarin and certain drugs used to treat diabetes, high cholesterol, stomach ulcers or high blood pressure.

Often other substances are added to curcumin supplements for certain reasons. Bromelain is sometimes added to increase the anti-inflammatory effect, however the majority of additives are included to increase bioavailability (the ability of your body to use the curcumin you take). Certain substances such as *piperine* increase the bioavailability of curcumin dramatically and thereby increasing the effectiveness of the dose you take. Curcumin has low bioavailability so if you are consuming, say, an Indian curry, your body is generally unable to take up much of the curcumin. In general, I like adding piperine supplements to my regime because many supplements (such as milk thistle) also suffer from low bioavailability. Alternatively, buy brands that combine the active agent with another substance (such as piperine) that increases bioavailability.

Curcumin for me is one of the most exciting supplements to come to prominence in recent times. Many herbs and supplements are either ineffective or too weak in comparison to any pharmaceutical options to be viable as treatments. Curcumin is no such supplement. Its effects are surprisingly potent – especially in the area of inflammation reduction. I believe inflammation is one of the largely undiagnosed epidemics of recent times, causing anything from cancer to heart disease.

There are not too many supplements out there that have positive effects on the brain, heart, liver, kidneys, stomach, joints and blood sugar. Curcumin is one such supplement.

Vitamin D

Vitamin D is another one that could be slotted into just about anywhere in this book. It is gradually become the nutritional version of the hottest Hollywood actor – everyone is talking about it. For years vitamin D was just that "thing" that people knew you "got from sunshine". However the latest research is indicating that Vitamin D is implicated a surprising array of health conditions that affect longevity.

However not only does vitamin D directly target inflammation, it also appears to directly target aging via inhibiting telomere shortening. It is believed to achieve this via its ability to inhibit pro-inflammatory processes. Vitamin D also inhibits certain kinds of dangerous cell proliferation mechanisms. For anyone out there with psoriasis, you would already be aware of this, as a vitamin D analogue called *calcipotriol* is a key ingredient in some anti-psoriasis creams, because it inhibits the cell proliferation associated with this particular skin condition.

A 2012 study which was published in the Journal of Immunology was able to clearly identify the cellular processes involved in vitamin D's inflammation-fighting abilities. The lead author concluded *"Patients with chronic inflammatory diseases, such as asthma, arthritis and prostate cancer, who are vitamin D deficient, may benefit from vitamin D supplementation to get their serum vitamin D levels above 30 nanograms/milliliter"*.

The latest recommendations are to get at least 20 minutes per day of direct sunlight on exposed sections of your body and to consider supplementing with vitamin D also. Remember that if you supplement with vitamin D, please ensure you also supplement with vitamin K to ensure that there are no cardiovascular complications from the extra vitamin D.

More controversial is the growing number of people who are experimenting with mega-doses of vitamin D. This goes against traditional advice regarding vitamin D toxicity, however some of these people are reporting startling improvements in a range of health complaints. It is too early to tell yet whether mega-dosing is a sensible practice, however what I can say with confidence is that the general recommendations for serum vitamin D levels and daily limits are too low. People such as the author of that particular book are consuming doses of vitamin D that doctors would consider toxic, yet are seeing a resolution of a range of illnesses. At the very least, this topic requires more research and a probable upwards revision of recommended daily levels.

When you visit the doctor to get a check-up and order certain tests, make sure you request a vitamin D test also. Some research suggests the majority of people in the western world are deficient due to avoidance of sunshine and changes in dietary habits from vitamin D-rich foods to grain-based junk food.

Prevent aging from sugar and AGEs

As we have already heard, AGEs are believed to play a central role in accelerated and premature cellular aging. So we therefore need to ensure we minimize consumption of AGEs or foods that trigger the production of AGEs. The single most powerful way to do this (and also address other factors in aging such as inflammation) is to minimize your consumption of sugar, and in particular, fructose. High levels of fructose consumption (and in particular, high-fructose corn syrup) promote both inflammation and the production of AGEs.

I like using extremes to illuminate potential issues with health and the best way to get an idea on why sugar ages you, we just have to look at what happens over time with diabetes. The elevated blood glucose levels associated with diabetes gradually ages and destroys parts of your body. The list of negative consequences of elevated blood sugar is long and extensive, however just a few of the problems include – diabetic neuropathy (where elevated blood glucose damages nerves), diabetic nephropathy (damage to kidneys from elevated blood sugar), diabetic retinopathy (damage to the retina from diabetes). From the same study published in *Nutrients* that I mentioned earlier in the book *"Accumulation of AGEs has been found in healthy aging persons, and this accumulation is higher during high glucose concentrations. Microvascular and macrovascular damage, seen in diabetes, is attributed to the accumulation of AGEs in tissues"*.

It's not the fat, but the 2.5 pounds of sugar that the average America consumes each week that is driving the obesity epidemic. This is because sugar (and other quick digesting carbohydrate bad-guys like bread and pasta) impair insulin and leptin sensitivity, directing your cells to store more energy as fat.

Put simply, if you want to get on top of inflammation, AGEs and the resultant acceleration of cellular aging, you have to minimize consumption of exogenous dietary AGEs and all forms of sugar.

One of the emerging theories on atherosclerosis and heart disease proposes that the formation of dangerous plaque in your arteries is largely causes by scarring caused as an unintended consequence of your immune system trying to neutralize AGEs.

Sugar is addictive and so dramatically cutting your consumption of sugar in a short space of time can result in all kinds of withdrawal effects, not unlike someone withdrawing from a street drug. Therefore, to maximize your chances of success, I suggest you gradually shift your diet away from sweeter flavors and back towards neutral or savory flavors.

The best example of this is sweetened beverages like coffee. Many people swear by the technique of gradually reducing the sugar you add to your hot drinks slowly enough so your taste buds don't notice. Like most people, when I was a child I could only tolerate tea or coffee with plenty of added sugar – a habit which usually carries over into adulthood for most. Nowadays, if I accidentally taste sweetened hot drinks, I find them intolerably sweet.

Your sense of taste tends to find a level of homeostasis based around your diet. If you consume a lot of sweets, you can tolerate sweeter food. If you eat a mainly savory diet, you tend to gravitate away from sweet food. The best way to see this in action is if you ever try a *ketogenic* diet for a few days. Ketogenic diets involve the consumption of almost no sweet foods or carbohydrates. In the absence of glucose, your body makes a kind of glucose proxy called *ketone bodies*, which your brain is able to use as a fuel source. The main benefit of this kind of diet is dramatic weight loss (again reinforcing why the best way to lose weight is to reduce carbohydrates and not fat). The interesting part happens when you reintroduce carbohydrates after the diet has ended. You will notice that a strange thing has happened to your taste buds – they have regained their sensitivity to sugar. Herein lies an extremely important point – if you find low-sugar diets difficult because you think you crave sweet flavours, you will soon adapt as your own taste buds adapt. Gradually, you will need less and less sugar to get that little mood-boost from foods on the sweet spectrum.

So what makes fructose so bad anyway? It all comes down to how your body processes fructose compared to glucose. Your body (and in particular, your brain) has a better ability to directly utilize glucose, whereas fructose must undergo a large proportion of its metabolism in the liver, where it is converted into free fatty acids, very low-density lipoprotein (VLDL – the type of cholesterol transporter that you *should* be worried about) and triglycerides. Not only are these substances known contributing factors for heart disease, they also tend to end up stored as fat.

Fructose has also been shown to interfere with leptin-mediated hunger signaling, making you feel less full and hungrier, which leads to greater weight accumulation.

It is one of the great modern-day tragedies that Americans have been subjected to the dietary horror that is *high-fructose corn syrup*. The American love affair with soda (which is largely sweetened with high-fructose corn syrup) is one of the major health emergencies facing its population.

Most Americans don't realize that in most other places around the world, high-fructose corn syrup is not widely used. Most countries sweeten commercially made products (such as sodas) using sucrose from cane sugar or sugar beets. For this, Americans have the good old USDA and Federal Government to thank. The various subsidies given to American farmers to grow corn, has led to frantic efforts to find uses for all this corn. This results in things like high-fructose corn syrup and ethanol fuel.

So for American readers, I need to add in another point. Learn to fastidiously read labels to look for high-fructose corn syrup. You may be horrified to find that most of the foods you enjoy are sweetened with corn syrup. A good option (if your budget allows) is to source from organic specialists like Whole Foods or Trader Joes, who tend to have better quality food available. Eventually, however, you may reach a conclusion which will open up a whole new world of healthy eating – your best option for reducing fructose (and therefore inflammation and AGEs, is to make more of your own food and reduce the amount of packaged food you consume.

One thing to note is that, as we stand now, there is considerable controversy as to exactly which foods either contain the most AGEs or trigger the production of AGEs in the body. For example, some believe butter to be high in a variant of AGEs, whereas others believe we should focus on sugar-related AGEs as being the most dangerous.

My position is that, until we get more research in on which foods to avoid, the no-brainer at the moment is to minimize fructose and in particular, avoid high-fructose corn syrup.

At this stage the only supplement with good research backing in terms of reducing the effects of AGEs is the vitamin B1 (thiamine) analog *benfotiamine*. Benfotiamine appears to reduce the damage associated with glycation and inhibits inflammation by modulating a protein known as *nuclear factor-kappaB* (NF-kB).

Identify and treat hypertension (high blood pressure)

It is almost redundant to include this section because throughout this book we are directly dealing with the majority of all the causes of high blood pressure. If you manage stress, reduce alcohol consumption and exercise regularly (all recommended here already), you significantly reduce your chances of developing hypertension.

Probably the only other major point missing from this book is reducing salt intake. The issue of salt intake is complicated because for the majority of the population, salt consumption is not a problem. Salt should really only be targeted when high blood pressure (that hasn't responded to the other dietary and behavioral recommendations) is an issue. For a while there, salt was becoming a kind of "bogeyman" (just like cholesterol was also) and the general population was making wholesale reductions to the amount of salt they consumed. The problem with this is that when you cut out one thing from your diet, you naturally increase another thing (unless you reduce the amount of food you consume, which is unlikely). This meant that broad-based salt reduction was followed by commensurate increases in the consumption of sugar and carbohydrate. That's fine if you have seriously high blood pressure, but not so great for someone with normal to low blood pressure.

Any book on increasing life expectancy must, either directly or indirectly, look at reducing your risk of dying from the major killers. High blood pressure is acknowledged as being one of the main causative factors in preventable death due to heart disease and stroke. The World Health Organization considers high blood pressure to be the number one preventable cause of death worldwide. This is why I need to include a section on high blood pressure. There are many other causes of early mortality that we don't yet have a clear, direct treatment for, such as certain cancers or neurological disease. Whereas with high blood pressure, just some simple lifestyle changes and in certain cases antihypertensive medication, can essentially remove this as a risk factor in your demise.

If you imagine a blocked garden hose turned on for a period of time, bulging in parts, you can also imagine why high blood pressure is such a massive problem. If high blood pressure is left untreated, you are at high risk for something eventually bursting – whether in the heart, brain or elsewhere in the cardiovascular system.

If you haven't already had your blood pressure tested, get it tested immediately. If your blood pressure is found to be on the high side, your doctor will either initially recommend lifestyle changes only, or they may be more cautious and want you to start taking an antihypertensive drug as well. This will particularly be the case if you have dangerously high blood pressure.

The beauty of treating high blood pressure is that it responds well to lifestyle changes and if that isn't enough, the drugs used are also considered relatively safe. The drugs used to treat high blood pressure are possibly the least controversial of all categories of medication. So, whereas we have a massive debate raging on the consequences of statin therapy for "high cholesterol" (inverted commas deliberate), antihypertensive drugs are considered almost universally safe. There are a few different categories, however depending on the doctor and the country you are in, you will most like be prescribed a thiazide diuretic, a calcium channel blocker, an ACE inhibitor or an adrenergic receptor antagonist (beta blockers and alpha blockers).

Don't be afraid to aggressively treat high blood pressure. There are few complications associated with low blood pressure (apart from dizziness-related problems), so it doesn't matter if your treatment overshoots your blood pressure a little to the low side.

However, as mentioned, if you follow the guidelines in this book regarding diet, exercise and stress-reduction, hypertension is unlikely except in cases where there is a strong genetic disposition.

Insulin and longevity

The media loves to use the word "epidemic" when describing anything. Most of the time this word is used to grab headlines and create click-bait. However if there is one thing that truly deserves the term, it is the current epidemic of type 2 diabetes in the western world.

Type 2 diabetes slowly destroys your body at the cellular level, leading to heart disease, diabetic retinopathy and kidney disease to name just a few conditions triggered by diabetes.

However many researchers have used the fact that type 2 diabetes can shorten life expectancy by 10 years or more as the basis for extensive research into the effects of high blood sugar and insulin resistance on general longevity.

Depending on the individual, they can either be insulin resistant, where there is sufficient insulin secreted however their cells aren't responding to the insulin (creating perpetually raised blood sugar) or they may have progressed to genuine type 2 diabetes where their insulin production is insufficient, leading to the same outcome – high blood sugar.

Both insulin and blood glucose are toxic when they remain elevated over a long period of time, stimulating the growth of tumors and damaging cell walls. The bad news is that as we age, almost everyone will display a certain degree of progressive insulin resistance.

The good news is that one of the most common drugs used to treat type 2 diabetes and insulin resistance, metformin, appears to provide a potent longevity promoting effect also in people without this condition. Some well-known experts in the field believe that *metformin may be the single most powerful longevity promoting drug available.*

One of the major benefits of caloric restriction (CR) is improved insulin responsiveness and it appears that metformin is able to mimic the beneficial effects of CR, without having to actually restrict calories. Considering I would rather poke my own eye out with a blunt stick rather than permanently go hungry, I see this as a massive benefit. Metformin appears to trigger the same gene expression associated with CR.

To name just a few of the benefits of metformin –

- Improved insulin sensitivity
- Lower LDL
- Increased levels of *AMP-activated protein kinase activity* (AMPK)[4]
- Increased antioxidant activity
- Reduced inflammation, as measured by CRP levels
- Reduced risk of cancer

---

[4] AMPK is associated with healthy glucose and fat metabolism and ensures sufficient energy production at the cellular level. The implication here is that metformin appears to address the other key component of longevity promotion – mitochondrial function

According to a recent study, the universally positive effects that metformin has in the body *"raise[s] the possibility of metformin-based interventions to promote healthy aging."*

There have been a range of studies using standard animal subjects including nematode worms and mice, with clear lifespan increasing effects observed. For example, the mice in the study who were given metformin, lived on average almost 6% longer than controls.

One of the interesting ways metformin promotes longevity is by inducing a form of mild oxidative stress. This appears to strengthen cells via hormetic mechanisms[5]. The result is, counterintuitively, less damaging oxidative stress in the long run. Researchers found that, in the case of metformin treatment, this "produced benefits, including reduced oxidative stress and increased antioxidant defenses, leading to lower oxidative damage accumulation and inhibition of chronic inflammation."

The net effect of metformin appears to be a restoration of your youthful insulin sensitivity.

However the good news doesn't end there. Researchers have discovered that by adding a prebiotic oligofructose supplement, subjects can achieve an even better improvement in insulin sensitivity than by just using metformin alone. You can get oligofructose in the form of a long chain *inulin* (not *insulin*, by the way – this is not a typo) supplement. Just look in the pre-biotics (not pro-biotics) section of your health food store or online supplement retailer.

Rather than viewing type 2 diabetes as a cause of premature aging, many experts view it as an *example* of premature aging. The key point is that type 2 diabetes should not be viewed as a genetic fait accompli. It is both preventable and it also serves as a diagnostic tool to monitor your own premature aging.

Naturally, metformin is a prescription drug that you will need to obtain from your doctor, who will only prescribe it to you if they were comfortable that it wouldn't create any problems or interact with other medication. For example, if you have impaired liver or kidney function metformin would be contraindicated. Some doctors are more across metformin than others. In fact, many doctors actually recommend all their patients over the age of 40 to take metformin, whether they are pre-diabetic or not.

Optimize liver function

As we have seen in the section on glutathione, a healthy liver is central to longevity as it is one of your front line defenses in detoxifying and repairing cellular damage. This organ bears the brunt of the modern lifestyle more than any other organ, as it is the liver that must deal with the consequences of a poor diet and the excess use of various drugs, medicines and alcohol.

Most people are aware of what is required to maintain a healthy heart and brain, however, apart from the general recommendation to "minimize alcohol consumption", the average person would struggle to list any of the other reasons a liver can become dysfunctional or any of the different substances which help to repair it.

---

[5] As mentioned elsewhere in this book, hormesis is the process by which you strengthen something by putting it under repeated, low level stress.

Outside of medical circles, almost no-one knows about *N-acetylcysteine and* hardly anyone knows about glutathione.

Ask the average person what the liver actually does, you will generally get either a blank look or a vague statement that *'it processes toxins'* or *'it cleans the blood'*. However, the liver does so much more. For example -

- The liver can create glucose (an important source of energy for your brain in particular) from glycogen, protein and fat

- The liver can create vital amino acids

- The liver creates the majority of all your cholesterol - yes - the amount of cholesterol in your blood is only weakly related to how much you consume via your diet!

- The liver creates triglyceride fats that your body can use for energy

- The liver produces certain substances which enable your blood to coagulate in the event of injury

- In the developing baby, before bone marrow is ready to assume the role, the liver is responsible for producing most of the baby's red blood cells

- The liver synthesizes and processes bile, which your body needs for digesting fats. Bile also facilitates the absorption of vitamin K from the diet. For anyone deficient in vitamin D or currently taking vitamin D supplements to correct a deficiency, vitamin K is incredibly important for ensuring that the body sends dietary calcium to your bones and not to your arteries.

- The liver produces *insulin-like growth factor 1* (IGF-1), a hormone which is hugely important to the natural development of children and continues to have an important role into adulthood.

- The liver breaks down various hormones after they are no longer required

- The liver processes bilirubin, one of the substances responsible for, how should I put this, your poop being brown.

- The liver is responsible for the majority of all drug metabolism. This can be either the processing of toxic substances (such as acetaminophen) or the conversion of a drug taken orally into a metabolite which is active in the body. For example, the popular painkiller codeine itself is virtually inactive; however in the liver, codeine is converted into morphine, a significantly more powerful drug. This is how codeine and similar drugs which require metabolism work.

- The liver converts toxic ammonia into urea via the urea cycle, to enable safe processing of this toxic substance

- The liver also acts as a storage house for a variety of vitamins and minerals including - vitamin A, vitamin D, vitamin B12, vitamin K, iron and copper.

- The liver, supporting the lymphatic system, is responsible for a healthy immune system via the production of various immunity-boosting substances

- The liver produces a hormone involved with regulating healthy blood pressure levels

So what can go wrong?

Hepatitis - this is the most common type of major liver disease, where inflammation of the liver is, except in rare cases, caused by the hepatitis virus.

Alcoholic liver disease - this is the catch-all term for liver diseases such as fatty liver, alcoholic hepatitis and cirrhosis which are all caused by the excess consumption of alcohol. Left untreated, these can lead to liver failure.

What are the symptoms of liver damage or a poorly functioning liver?

- Pale stools - sorry to bring up poop again. Remember bilirubin I just mentioned which gives poop its brown tint? A damaged liver doesn't produce enough of it so pale stools can eventuate

- Dark colored urine

- Jaundice, where the skin or the whites of the eyes can take on a yellow tint. This is because of the poorly functioning liver's inability to correctly process bilirubin, leading to its deposit in the skin

- Abdominal swelling, indigestions, acid reflux and fat-soluble vitamin deficiencies caused by the inability to properly absorb fat

- Fatigue caused by a lack of nutrients and hormones produced by the liver

- Excessive bruising or bleeding due to a lack of that substance I mentioned that enables blood to clot

- A poorly functioning liver can also impact your brain and nervous system, leading to mood changes (particularly depression) and an inability to concentrate.

- Elevated cholesterol levels

If you suspect that you have a poorly functioning liver, before you do anything, visit your doctor and request liver function tests. These tests look for certain enzymes which are associated with the liver. Abnormal levels of these enzymes can point to a potential issue with liver function.

The good news is that the liver has an unequalled ability to regenerate itself. Your liver is an amazing organ which can take most of what life throws at it. Imagine if you cut three-quarters of your finger off and it grew back. This is what the liver is capable of. Under certain circumstances, a person could regrow a new liver from only around a quarter of a normal liver.

This means that, for a person with a healthy diet, who does not take a large amount of legal or illegal drugs (including medicines), who does not consume a large amount of alcohol and who doesn't have any pre-existing genetic or lifestyle related liver disease, you have absolutely no need to be concerned. However, the problem is that many people do drink excessive quantities of alcohol, take illicit drugs, use a variety of medications and follow a poor diet.

The other piece of good news is that the liver responds dramatically to certain supplements. If someone has issues with a poorly functioning liver, through the use of certain supplements, they will see quite dramatic improvements in functioning and reap the consequent longevity-related benefits.

Out of all the various supplements which are promoted for a healthy liver, only four meet my criteria in having solid scientific backing through clinical trials -

- **N-Acetylcysteine (NAC)**
- **Milk thistle (silymarin)**
- **Curcumin**
- **Alpha lipoic acid (ALA)**

Are you starting to see a pattern here?

I have covered NAC, ALA and curcumin in the sections on glutathione and inflammation, so I just need to now cover what is probably the single most powerful liver optimizing supplement available - *milk thistle*.

However I should point out that one of the key ways in which milk thistle heals the liver is the same as the other supplements covered - it increases levels of glutathione.

When I first heard of milk thistle a few years ago, I was initially quite skeptical about claims regarding the ability to detoxify and rejuvenate the liver. Well, I was wrong. Subsequent research uncovered an amazing amount of research on this fascinating herb. The research is unequivocal – milk thistle really does repair the liver.

Milk thistle has been used for 2000 years as natural treatment for various diseases such as kidney, cancer and gall bladder problems, lowering cholesterol levels, hepatitis B and C, spleen disorders, malaria, menstrual problems and swelling of the lungs. It is extracted from the seeds (fruit) of the milk thistle plant and the seeds are used to prepare capsules, extracts, powders, and tinctures. Now, just because something has been used for certain conditions for thousands of years, that doesn't mean that it has been proven to work for those conditions. To prove that something works, you need to conduct randomized, double-blind placebo controlled trials. As I will soon show, it is in these trials that milk thistle has shone.

When we talk about milk thistle as a supplement, in general what we are talking about is a single phenol called *silymarin*, which the milk thistle is high in. If you want to get even more specific, the active constituent of silymarin is called *silibinin (or silibin)*, a flavonoid with powerful antioxidant actions. When you purchase milk thistle as a supplement, in general you are purchasing a standardized extract of silymarin.

Milk thistle has solid evidence backing its use for –

- Repairing liver damage caused by overuse of medications, alcohol and street drugs

- Improving life expectancy for patients with cirrhosis of the liver

- Assisting in the treatment of viral hepatitis

- Preventing acute liver damage from ingesting high doses of hepatotoxic (toxic to the liver) substances such as acetaminophen and Death Cap Mushroom

- Assisting in the treatment of mild depression

- Milk Thistle appears to increase bile solubility, potentially demonstrating benefit in preventing or treating gallstones.

One of the best ways to view milk thistle without getting bogged down in too much detail, is to think of it as a super-potent antioxidant. Milk thistle hunts down free radicals which have been shown to damage cells and accelerate certain aspects of the aging process. Milk Thistle not only acts as an antioxidant itself but also increases the activity of other antioxidants such as *superoxide dismutase*, which we know to be an incredibly powerful fighter of oxidative damage.

However, one of the most interesting aspects of milk thistle is that it has been shown to increase levels of glutathione in the liver by significant amounts, like NAC and ALA.

Milk thistle also acts as an anti-inflammatory by inhibiting levels of *leukotriene*, a pro-inflammatory substance that has been linked to everything from heart disease to cancer to psoriasis.

So, milk thistle repairs the liver, increases glutathione and reduces inflammation. You can see why I initially struggled to work out exactly *where* in this book I should cover this interesting herb.

As you would imagine from a substance that acts as an antioxidant, milk thistle has some solid research backing regarding its anti-cancer properties. Now, whenever I read 'natural therapy' and 'cancer' I immediately get suspicious. Too many times I have heard of a cancer patient refusing chemotherapy to try something like homeopathy, which I strongly oppose. When you are diagnosed with cancer, it is not the time to abandon modern western medicine. However, surprisingly, not only has the anti-cancer action of milk thistle been demonstrated, so has the mechanism by which it acts.

One of the most promising areas of research into a potential cure for cancer has been looking at the blood vessels which feed cancers and thereby allowing them to grow. If you can cut of the blood supply to cancers, you can stop them from spreading. Incredibly, milk thistle has shown to possess exactly this property. Now, let me be clear however – this in no way means that milk thistle can currently be viewed as a viable alternative to pharmaceutical drugs for the treatment of advanced cancers. However, what it does show is a clear mechanism for inhibiting the growth and spread of early cancers. To put it another way, milk thistle could prove to be a useful supplement for those who want to reduce their risk of getting a deadly cancer by stopping early cancers in their tracks. So far, milk thistle has demonstrated the ability to fight prostate, skin, ovarian, colon, breast, lung and cervical cancers.

A 2007 study found that an extract of milk thistle blocked hepatitis C virus (HCV) cell culture infection of human hepatoma cultures. Another study conducted in 2010 found that the eight major compounds that comprise milk thistle, including seven flavonolignans and one flavonoid are all inhibitors of HCV RNA-dependent RNA polymerase.

According to a study published in the journal *Phytotherapy Research* in 2006, milk thistle may also keep insulin levels more stable by regulating or decreasing the blood glucose levels in the body. This is interesting for two reasons – not just the obvious benefits for patients with type 2 diabetes. Insulin is also heavily implicated in weight gain via fat accumulation in the body – particularly around the belly for males. This implies potential uses for milk thistle in the area of weight management. However the evidence at this stage is only preliminary so I wouldn't recommend going out and buying milk thistle to lose weight.

A study also showed that the flavonoid component of milk thistle helped to lower cholesterol and triglyceride levels, which are often high in people who are overweight or obese. High levels of fats in the blood can also lead to increased risk of cardiovascular disease. Triglyceride levels in particular are becoming more and more implicated as one of the key risk factors in heart disease. The ability of fish oil (omega 3 fatty acids) to decrease the risk of heart disease is due in no small part by the ability of fish oil to decrease levels of triglycerides in the blood.

Another case report points to a potential indirect use for milk thistle in the fight against cancer. A woman who was suffering from a type of leukemia was given Milk Thistle extract while being treated with powerful immunosuppressive and steroidal drugs. This patient had required regular treatment breaks due to adverse changes in liver enzyme levels. After treatment with Milk Thistle, the patient's liver enzymes normalized and she was able to continue treatment without further interruption. Naturally this is only a case report, not a clinical trial, however it points to a potential use for milk thistle to maintain a healthy liver when it is being assaulted by potent drugs needed to either cure a cancer patient or extend life expectancy. Fortunately, this potential application for milk thistle has been backed up with a clinical trial.

In this promising double-blind, placebo-controlled trial, a group children who were receiving treatment for acute lymphoblastic leukemia were unfortunately showing signs of hepatotoxicity (liver damage) caused by their chemotherapy drugs. The children were split into two groups with one group receiving milk thistle extract and the other group a placebo. The results of the trial were that the group receiving milk thistle extract showed significantly lower levels of *alanine aminotransferase* than the placebo group. Alanine aminotransferase is a reliable indicator of liver damage, so this result was extremely encouraging and further backed up the previous case report.

Another randomized controlled trial supported by the *National Institute of Diabetes and Digestive and Kidney Diseases* involved patients with hepatitis C who had not responded to antiviral therapy. The study involved assessing all the various herbal medicines and natural therapies to ascertain whether there was any benefit. Out of those taking herbal supplements, over 70% involved milk thistle extract. Patients were surveyed regarding all aspects of their health and wellbeing. The study found that those patients taking milk thistle extract showed significantly fewer adverse symptoms and enjoyed a much higher quality of life. This is extremely encouraging however I should point out that these studies that involve subjects self-reporting are notoriously unreliable. It is very easy to convince yourself that you have better quality of life because you are taking milk thistle – it is much harder to influence levels of alanine aminotransferase by placebo effect alone.

Another report mentions milk thistle as the only effective antidote in patients with liver damage from Death Cap Mushroom (*Amanita Phalloides*) poisoning. Patients received doses of milk thistle extract, which demonstrated clear effectiveness in preventing the liver damage associated with this type of poisoning. Again, the other benefit was that there were no reports of adverse events or side-effects. Naturally, unless you are particularly unlucky, having the antidote for Death Cap Mushroom poisoning has little to do with longevity. However it does give an indication of the potent actions of milk thistle in the body.

However the best kind of clinical trial data comes from meta-analyses, which is where all the results from different trials are put together to create an overall picture of a certain medication or supplement. The two main meta-analyses which have been conducted on Milk Thistle have been a *Cochrane Review* in 2005 and an *Agency for Healthcare Research and Quality* (AHRQ) study. Both of these reviews reached a similar conclusion – that whilst the data on milk thistle for treating diseases of the liver were encouraging, many of the studies were poorly designed and that the actual mechanism by which milk thistle works is still a little unclear. This doesn't mean that they believed milk thistle didn't work, just that it had not yet been proven to the degree to which they would feel comfortable recommending this herb as a front-line treatment for liver diseases.

The Cochrane Review looked at thirteen randomized clinical trials which assessed milk thistle in 915 patients with alcoholic and/or Hepatitis B or C. They concluded that whilst there appeared to be some beneficial effects, there was still a lack of evidence to recommend milk thistle on a widespread basis.

One of the problems with milk thistle, like curcumin, it its low level of bioavailability. What this means is that even though you are taking a potentially large dose, much of it is not absorbed by your body. Recently there has been two fantastic developments in efforts to improve absorption and therefore effectiveness. Firstly, scientists have identified more clearly that silibin is the main active constituent of milk thistle and have subsequently produced purified versions with only silibin. This increases the potency and therefore the ability of the body to absorb enough to obtain the desired benefits. Secondly, a new phospholipid complex call *Siliphos* has been developed. Siliphos is essentially silibin bound with soy-based phospholipids to improve the body's ability to absorb the silibin. This results in dramatically increased levels of silibin in the blood after administration, compared to standard silibin supplementation.

Milk thistle appears to be surprisingly free of any serious adverse effects considering how potently it acts in the body. For some people it can have a mild laxative effect and in massive overdose is can cause nausea, stomach pain, vomiting, headaches, joint pain, indigestion, itching, bloating and diarrhea. However I should point out that you would need to consume a massive dose to see anything like this.

As with just about any supplement, pregnant women should avoid milk thistle as there is no conclusive evidence proving lack of harm (or harm for that matter) at this stage. Any potential liver boosting effects of milk thistle should be put to one side when you are pregnant.

Due to the lack of adverse effects and dangers, there is little requirement for highly specialized or specific dosages, however in general you could target between 400-800mg per day in divided doses.

If you are currently suffering from a diagnosed liver disease such as alcoholic cirrhosis or hepatitis, milk thistle should be an almost automatic option alongside your conventional therapies. As a repairer of your liver, milk thistle is without equal in the herbal world.

However if you are currently relatively healthy but are worried about liver health or put your liver under a lot of strain from alcohol and drugs, I believe you should also make milk thistle one of your front line options for keeping your liver in great condition. People forget that their liver is up there with the heart and brain in terms of importance for your survival. It is involved in so many different functions in the body that that keeping it in the best condition possible should be a priority for anyone looking towards maximizing their own longevity.

Virus-based gene therapy

A potential prelude to widespread gene therapy to prevent premature aging is being offered by a company based in South America. The company, Bioviva, uses benign viruses to deliver targeted gene therapy which implants telomerase at a specific location in your DNA. Yes you read that correctly. They inject viruses in you as an anti-aging therapy.

This kind of therapy is right at the cutting edge and therefore not widely available yet. However the initial results have been extremely encouraging.

The viruses, which are known as adeno-associated viruses (AAV), insert the therapeutic genetic material into a targeted location on chromosome 19. These viruses are harmless in humans and lack the ability to replicate. They appear to optimize telomerase function, which leads to longer telomeres and consequently, increased longevity.

As we are talking genuinely cutting edge here, anyone receiving therapy is, at least to some degree, a potential guinea pig. However, based on current evidence, this therapy appears to be safe.

The reason why it is being offered in Mexico and Columbia (and not the US) is that the therapy is not yet FDA-approved. If and when the FDA approves this kind of therapy, it may become more widely available. Until then it remains available only to those who are flush with cash and who don't have the luxury of waiting for FDA approval.

Nicotinamide adenine dinucleotide (NAD+)

Among the compounds and drugs being developed to fight aging, despite not being widely available, NAD+ is one of the most promising angles. NAD+ is central to the production of energy at the cellular/mitochondrial level and levels appear to naturally decline as we age. This decline in NAD+ is believed to be one of the major contributors to the process of cellular aging and has therefore been the main target of several biotech companies who have been developing therapies to boost NAD+.

NAD+ is a vital co-factor in the production and maintenance of sirtuins and boosting NAD+ appears to mitigate sirtuin-mediated cellular aging. This is the same pathway targeted by resveratrol supplementation, however, whereas resveratrol has demonstrated only weak ability to modulate sirtuin activity, NAD+ appears to do this in a more direct and potent way. Or to put it another way, NAD+ appears to confer all the benefits of caloric restriction, without the requirement to starve yourself. In essence, by engaging in caloric restriction, you are trying to boost NAD+, which then positively influences sirtuin activity. However there appears to be ways of doing this more directly.

Currently, the most promising option is a form of vitamin B3 called nicotinamide riboside (NR). NR appears to deactivate one of the key drivers of premature aging, leading to increased longevity and cognitive functions. To be honest, the animal trials to date seem almost too good to be true. In various animals, from mice to worms, NR leads to significant increases in longevity. In mice fed an extremely high fat diet, NR-treated mice gained less weight than the control mice, had significantly better endurance and showed improved insulin sensitivity. In the brain, NR appears to prevent neurodegeneration by repairing and protecting a key part of the neuron which is vital for communication between brain cells.

A trial on mice conducted by Harvard researcher Doctor David Sinclair found that supplementing NR restored the two-year old mouse's mitochondria to that of a six month old mouse. In humans, this corresponds to restoring a 60 year old person's mitochondria to the equivalent of a 20 year old person.

This is not fringe research either. Both MIT and the Mayo Clinic are currently investigating the potential of NR to treat conditions as diverse as heart disease and Alzheimer's. A recent study published in EMBO Molecular Medicine found that –

> *"Oral administration of nicotinamide riboside (NR), a vitamin B3 and NAD+ precursor, was previously shown to boost NAD+ levels in mice and to induce mitochondrial biogenesis. Here, we treated mitochondrial myopathy mice with NR. This vitamin effectively delayed early- and late-stage disease progression, by robustly inducing mitochondrial biogenesis in skeletal muscle and brown adipose tissue, preventing mitochondrial ultrastructure abnormalities and mtDNA deletion formation. NR further stimulated mitochondrial unfolded protein response, suggesting its protective role in mitochondrial disease. These results indicate that NR and strategies boosting NAD+ levels are a promising treatment strategy for mitochondrial myopathy."*

If you are interested in NR, the good news is that it has recently become available from a few different sources. Interestingly, one of these products, called "Basis", contains not only NR, but a more recently discovered, super-potent alternative to resveratrol, known as pterostilbene. Pterostilbene, which is found naturally in blueberries, is a nearly identical molecule to resveratrol, but overcomes resveratrol's unfortunate lack of bioavailability. Pterostilbene theoretically works synergistically with NR to restore mitochondrial function.

As more and more early adopters experiment with these NAD+ boosters, it will be very interesting to see what kinds of effects we see in humans. Unless you have a pressing need to restore mitochondrial function, perhaps the smartest thing would be to sit back and wait to see the results of more real world results and human clinical trials.

Exercise

Exercise is the single greatest thing you can do for your brain. And evolution knows it too, which is why there is a complex system of biochemical reactions that reward you when you exercise.

You have probably heard of the *runner's high* right? You have probably also heard that this "high" comes from endorphins, your body's own internal morphine. Well, it turns out that this is only partly true. But I'll get to that in a bit.

In terms of building a super-brain, the single most important factor is relating to BDNF (*brain-derived neurotrophic factor*), your brain's own "*miracle-gro*" (as I have heard a few other authors refer to it as). BDNF is a protein that helps your existing brain cells to thrive and also helps drive important aspects of neurogenesis – the birth of new neurons. Neurogenesis seems so commonplace nowadays that it is easy to forget that up until only a few years ago it was believed that neurogenesis was impossible. Remember being told that you are born with a certain number of brain cells and can never grow new ones? Well, it turns out that was incorrect.

It also turns out that exercise is the single most powerful behaviour you can engage in to stimulate the secretion of BDNF in important parts of the brain such as the hippocampus. The hippocampus is central to a sharp brain (particularly memory recall) and a good mood. The hippocampus of depressed people is often found to have actually shrunk by a measurable amount! The good news is that, of all the areas in your brain, the hippocampus is one of the best at recovering and growing new neurons.

In terms of exercise for neural functioning, there is a great body of work centered on dementia patients, such as those with Alzheimer's. As I often mention, research on Alzheimer's gives us great indications regarding what works to improve cognition and memory.

Therefore, it is unsurprising that multiple studies have shown that exercise improves aspects of dementia both acutely and chronically. What this means is that a single episode of exercise (say, jogging for 30 minutes) increases production of BDNF and improves markers of cognition (acutely), while a continued exercise program gives additional benefits which gradually accumulate (chronically).

However it is in the area of depression and anxiety treatment that exercise has the most research behind it.

In his book Spark!: How exercise will improve the performance of your brain, John Ratey cites study after study which clearly demonstrates the link between exercise and not only mood, but cognitive function also. If you are serious about understanding the nexus between exercise and brain health, I strongly urge you to read books such as Ratey's. He was trying to get the message out about this important topic before anyone else – a true trailblazer.

As I mentioned in the introduction to this section, for quite a few years now the accepted wisdom was that runner's high was caused by endorphins. In fact, it's hard to believe that only a few years before that, we still had no idea about the existence of your body's own internal "morphine". For years scientists wondered why exactly was it that your brain had its own locks (opiate receptors) which morphine and other opiates (the keys) perfectly fit. Eventually endorphins (literally "endogenous morphine") were discovered as being the natural painkilling chemical produced by your body in times of stress or physical pain.

So that perfectly explains why you feel good when you exercise and why exercise treats depression right? As with anything to do with the brain, it is a little more complicated.

There is a drug called *naloxone* which completely neutralizes the effects of opiates on the brain. If you take naloxone and then shoot heroin, you don't get high. Which is why it is often a component of addiction treatment. It turns out that if you give someone naloxone and then they exercise, the naloxone only negates some aspects of the mood boost you get from exercise.

Subsequent research on both animals and humans has shown that exercise also increases levels of your *monoamines* – serotonin, dopamine and norepinephrine. Yes, exercising really is like popping a happy pill.

Exercise also improves oxygenation of the brain through improved blood flow. Your brain is a massive oxygen and energy sponge, so anything which improves delivery of this vital fuel to where it's needed is going to be hugely beneficial.

Finally, exercise also helps in an indirect way by improving one of the most important aspects of brain health – sleep. Sleep is where your brain does the majority of its repair work – particularly during *slow wave sleep* (stage 3 & 4 "NREM" sleep) which is your deepest stage of sleep.

As you probably know, while you are asleep, your brain goes through various stages which can all be measured with a polysomnograph. You are probably most familiar with one of these stages – REM ("rapid eye movement") sleep. Slow wave sleep is when the majority of your brain's repair work happens. Exercise increases slow wave sleep, meaning that not only do you wake more refreshed than you would otherwise be, but your brain has been able to accelerate its repair work.

There is still some debate as to why exercise helps with sleep quality and quantity. I believe that it is a combination of factors. Firstly, exercise burns off a lot of stress hormones and neurotransmitters such as cortisol and norepinephrine, leading to increased relaxation and deeper sleep – you sleep much more lightly when you are stressed or physiologically aroused. Secondly, exercise, when done in the late a f t e r n o o n particularly, artificially raises your core body temperature. Scientists still aren't sure why, but raising your body temperature a few hours before bed will increase slow wave sleep. This is the reason why hot baths before bed also increase slow wave sleep. The cooling that happens as your body slides down into sleep, appears to set off some kind of biochemical reaction that leads to better sleep quality.

So, if we acknowledge that exercise super-charges your brain and improves your mood, the next question is – *What kind of exercise?*

My philosophy is always to focus on doing what you enjoy. If you force yourself to do something you hate, you will soon give up and be back at square one. If you hate jogging, don't try to force yourself to jog. Be guided by how you feel. After reading so often about how jogging before breakfast accelerates weight loss, I decided to force myself to jog as soon as I woke up. It only took me a few times before I realized I hated it so much that I would never keep it up. However, come 11am each morning, I love nothing better than to hit the gym or even go for the occasional run.

Ideally you will be doing a mixture of – cardiovascular exercise, strength training and stretches. I am a massive fan of H.I.I.T (*high intensity interval training*) for brain health. I am also a busy, impatient guy, so I love to get my exercise done quickly. So don't think that you need to spend an hour on a treadmill. You could literally find a grassed area and do, say, 5 x 100 meter sprints and you would see massive benefits for your brain. It could be all over in 10 minutes. There is a whole new science emerging recently which supports the idea that the best kind of exercise is short in duration and high intensity.

Pick what you love and just keep at it. Remember, one of the mainstays of depression treatment is walking. Yes, just getting out of the house and walking at a leisurely pace can have a dramatic effect on symptoms of depression.

Get socially connected

We humans are social animals. We have evolved to form deep bonds with a community of friends and family around us. Some evolutionary psychologists have even hypothesized that the reason we needed to develop such a complex and powerful brain (in my case this is debatable) was to manage a complex web of co-operative relationships with those around us.

One of the easiest ways to see this is to consider what happens when people become isolated. In general, if we are separated from loved ones or even from any human being at all, we become depressed and occasionally our grasp on reality can even unravel.

In his landmark book "The Blue Zones: Lessons for Living Longer from people who lived the longest", author Dan Buettner identified certain locations around the world that are characterized by an unusually high number of centenarians. They were - Okinawa (Japan), Sardinia (Italy), Nicoya (Costa Rica), Icaria (Greece) and a group of Seventh Day Adventists in Loma Linda, California.

After identifying these longevity superstars, the most important point should be identifying why these populations live longer and healthier lives. Each of these areas had their own unique tendencies which were believed to be contributing factors. So for example, the Loma Linda Seventh Day Adventists ate plenty of nuts, whereas the Sardinians drank polyphenol-rich red wine.

Where this line of inquiry got really interesting however, was when researchers looked for unifying factors that held consistent across all of these "blue zones". In the below Venn diagram you can see that these common traits were - emphasis on family, no smoking, regular physical activity, social engagement and the consumption of legumes.

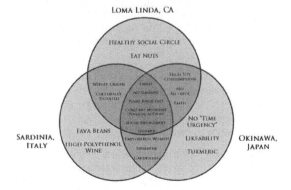

(Chart source: Wikipedia)

I have to admit being surprised to see legumes in there, considering the range of nutritional shortcomings they have. My first instinct is to think that legumes are there mainly by chance - I think it is correlation not causation. However I am also prepared to accept the possibility that there is something as yet unidentified regarding the health benefits of legumes. One thing is for certain however - legumes are not sending these people to an early grave, so perhaps we need to do more study into this vegetarian staple.

So, the thing that immediately sticks out is the fact that two of the unifying factors in the blue zones are "family" and "social engagement", which I would argue are one and the same in terms of coming under the general umbrella of *socialization promoting longevity*.

As I have spent an improbably large amount of time recently researching longevity and the factors that promote it, the importance of maintaining social connections is the single, unchanging factor. Some groups that are long lived eat plenty of fish, while others are mainly vegetarian. Some drink no alcohol, whereas others drink red wine. However all of them maintain a rich network of social and familial ties. Or to put it another way, when different groups are studied, no one ever cites "isolation and loneliness" as a factor in their longevity.

To learn the importance of social ties for a person's longevity, it is helpful to look at what goes wrong in your brain and body when you are isolated.

Fortunately, in the area of neuroscience and mental health, there is a large body of work we can draw from when looking at the brain of a lonely, isolated person. Isolation is a potent trigger for mood disorders, leading to various changes in the brain and cardiovascular system.

Study into the effects of isolation on the human mind can be traced back to renowned psychotherapist Frieda Fromm-Reichmann. Reichmann's seminal 1959 work *"On Loneliness"* is considered the starting point of modern-day loneliness studies. This has led to a variety of studies into the neurobiological effect of isolation and loneliness. One particular study showed that a lack of social interaction as a young animal (whether a human or a rodent) had enduring negative effects on the human brain such as dysfunctional myelin sheaths (the fatty tubes that protect the axon component of a neuron). Functional myelin are vital for normal nerve transmission, as we can see from the progressive neurological disease multiple sclerosis, which is caused by auto-immune medicated destruction of myelin.

Also, isolation leads to chronically lowered levels of the feel-good neurotransmitter serotonin. It is one of the bizarre ironies of major depression that being depressed causes people to withdraw from the most powerful antidepressant known - rich and varied social contact. However therein lies a rich lesson also - in some cases one of the quickest and most effective ways to reverse depression is to socialize.

Isolation appears to be particularly lethal for the elderly, accelerating the rate at which cognition and memory declines. And this is not just rare occurrences either. A 2010 survey in the US found that more than a third of elderly people consider themselves to be "chronically lonely". Any broad-based effort by government to promote longevity or the health of the elderly, must, by definition, pay particular attention to alleviating this chronic loneliness. There are many things we can do as a society to ensure that the elderly don't live out their days in a level of isolation that is hastening their demise. Perhaps we can redirect certain community service activities away from picking up rubbish or cleaning graffiti off walls and back towards spending quality time with the elderly.

One thing we must be careful of, however, is to avoid applying blanket generalizations to what is a diverse group of people on the planet. We must refrain from defining loneliness purely in terms of physical isolation from other human beings. It is possible for certain people to spend their life at various cocktail parties and shindigs, yet feel interminably lonely. There must be a connection between the person and the environment. If you forced a shy, socially anxious person to spend their life at dinner parties, you would possibly be harming them, not helping. Not only do we need to differentiate between natural extroverts and natural introverts, we need to differentiate between someone who is an introvert and someone who is pathologically shy. As Susan Cain points out in her brilliant book Quiet: The power of introverts in a world that can't stop talking, there is a difference between the two and the key word is "pathological". Being an introvert is not necessarily pathological, whereas being painfully shy is.

So whether you are applying this concept for yourself or whether we are looking at broad measures to increase longevity via social interaction, we need to account for variations in personality. This is extremely challenging however. If you are reading this now and you tend to be introverted, do you have a clear idea whether forcing yourself to socialize would be beneficial or not? My advice would be that if you are depressed and alone, you have nothing to lose by forcing yourself to socialize. If for some reason you find it distressing and believe it may be exacerbating your condition, then by all means stop. However I tend to believe that genuine introverts who thrive in isolation are exceedingly rare. By nature, I tend to isolate myself and withdraw into my own little world. However, when I spend certain periods doing a lot of socialization, it does give a noticeable mood boost. I am not particularly beset by bad moods often, however I have noticed on many occasions I was in a bad mood and was dreading an upcoming social engagement (slightly lowered serotonin driving my urge to withdraw?), yet when I started talking to people at the party (or whatever it was) my mood would noticeably brighten in quite dramatic fashion.

You are fighting a lot of evolutionary force by isolating yourself. Evolution (if you could give it humanoid desires) really, really wants you to socialize. Humans are relatively weak if you compare us to the other predators that were prowling the African savannah. What has set us apart throughout history has been our ability to co-operate. Whether we are co-operating to bring down a large prey animal, building huts, protecting the tribe or raising children, it has been this factor which most evolutionary biologists cite as a key difference between man and even our nearest primate relatives.

Throughout human evolution, isolating yourself has not been a good idea at all. You were likely to either starve or be eaten in short order. So your biology sends you strong messages to create multitudinous co-operative and emotional connections with other humans. Just like your brain gives you liberal spurts of dopamine to reward you for finding high-calorie food or a potential mate, your brain sends you a strong message as if to say *Hey you. Get out there and make connections with people. I am withholding all this sweet, sweet serotonin until you do so.*

One thing we need to take into consideration however, is that a lack of social contact possibly makes us feel bad because of conditioned connotations as well. Society can generalize loneliness or isolation as being "sad" - hence the expression "sad & lonely". So are we sad because isolation is inherently depressing or because we are conditioned to think it is so? I tend to still think there is something neurobiological at work, because of what we have seen with rodent tests. Rodents are not brought up to think that "alone" should equal "sad".

However, if we look to meditative contemplatives we can see that with extensive training, sometimes this reaction can be retrained. Over the last few thousand years, Buddhist monks, Indian yogis and other adepts of contemplative traditions have institutionalized the practice of spending large chunks of time in complete isolation. Tibetan lamas, for example, have a tradition of retiring to a cave somewhere for months of meditation with no human contact.

While beginners who try extended period of secluded meditation can risk triggering psychosis or other mental illness, advanced meditators emerge from these periods enveloped in a kind of supernatural bliss. So why are these select few able to run counter to our understanding of socialization's effects on mood and longevity? Extended periods of isolation are characterized by an intense awareness of both the internal world and each word of what must seem like an endless monologue. Perhaps their practice of mindfulness allows them to take the emotional sting out of this incessant chatter? I don't know for sure, however it points to an interesting area of future research because, if we can identify exactly what is the difference between these people and ourselves, we may be able to create targeted future therapies.

I imagine that there are various evolutionary reasons why face to face socializing is more effective, however you also need to be pragmatic. Perhaps you are particularly socially anxious or live in an isolated part of the world. Use the internet to connect, whether through dating sites, social networks or gaming communities. Each time you type something and something comes back from another human, that's a connection.

Also, it could be of use to practice mindfulness, emulating our meditative contemplatives. Mindfulness therapy for mood disorders is one of the fastest growing sub-types of modern-day cognitive behavioral therapy. By practicing mindfulness, perhaps you are able to mitigate isolation as a possible causative factor in a shortened life-span.

However, at the end of the day, the beauty of socialization as a longevity-enhancing strategy is that your single act of connecting with someone socially has the ability to set off a beneficial chain reaction. The most obvious example is our previous example of someone keeping a lonely elderly person company. This act creates two "longevity units" (a completely made-up word by the way) concurrently. Your longevity is enhanced by both the social connection and the self-esteem boost you will get from doing something seemingly altruistic. The elderly person's longevity is also increased by a certain number of "longevity units" (you could argue that they get more units because at their age they would expect to get more noticeable benefit from social connections).

Where this gets truly interesting is where your increased socialization sets off a chain reaction. If we acknowledge that happier people socialize more (both as cause and effect, it goes both ways), then surely there is the likelihood that your act leads to other people socializing more as well. It has the potential to go on endlessly.

All the antioxidants in the world won't offset the life-span shortening effects of isolation. It needs to be a priority.

Reduce stress

If I told you that stress will send you to an early grave, it wouldn't be particularly surprising right? What about if I also told you that stress would also help you to live longer? Surely they can't both be correct can they?

The key is to specify the type of stress. There is a beneficial type called *eu*stress and the more pernicious type known as *di*stress. Eustress is the occasional stressful event that pushes you to achieve a goal or overcome a challenge. This is the kind of stress for which you are evolutionarily prepared - stressful event followed by action, followed by resolution. Distress is the problem. When we refer to stress, we are usually referring to distress.

Your body is singularly unprepared for the type of chronic, unrelenting stress that often typifies modern life. Think about the tyrant boss, for example. Your brain and endocrine system has no correlate from which to draw from in order to deal effectively with this kind of stress.

It is for this reason that stress is such a noxious aspect of modern life, hastening the demise of far too many people. If we just look at cardiovascular related deaths alone and consider the proportion of those where high blood pressure was a causative factor, and consider the role that stress plays in high blood pressure (hypertension), stress must be considered one of the major causes of premature death.

Chronic stress is ruinous for the human body and brain. One of the main problems is the chronically elevated levels of the glucocorticoid hormone *cortisol* that stress causes. Cortisol is hugely important for many functions. Cortisol helps you wake up each morning (it waxes and wanes appropriately in sympathy with your circadian rhythm) and helps you to deal with acutely stressful events. The problems start to occur when stress is unrelenting and cortisol remains elevated for long periods of time.

Cortisol is particularly toxic for your hippocampus, the part of your brain responsible for a range of functions linked to memory recall and context detection. Even in a test tube, cortisol damages hippocampal neurons. It is therefore unsurprising that chronic stress is a known causative factor in dementia, where years of elevated cortisol has gradually impaired the hippocampus.

However the damage is not just isolated to the brain and cardiovascular system. Chronically elevated cortisol is responsible for, or implicated in, a litany of health problems including - insulin resistance, impaired immune system, type 2 diabetes, fat around the belly (in men), decreased bone density and libido problems.

The solution, however, is not to lock yourself in a padded room to avoid any possible source of stress. As I mentioned a moment ago, certain types of acute stress are actually good for you as they help you achieve goals or avoid danger.

Regular but brief stressful episodes are also important as they make you stronger via the process of *hormesis*. In biology, hormesis refers to a small dose of something conferring consequent increased levels of resistance to that particular stressor. In one sense, this is just a fancy was of saying - *what doesn't kill you will make you stronger*. The most common example of this is a vaccine, where you get a small, survivable dose of something infectious or dangerous and are then immune to it from that point on.

So please don't create a form of chronic stress by worrying about occasional acute stress. That occasional stress of the upcoming presentation or the final exam is good for you in most cases.

However, there are a few complicating factors.

Firstly, each of us has a different reaction to stress. Stress is cumulative. When researchers have studied cases of major depression they found something interesting. In a large number of cases, there was a gradual accumulation of stressful experiences which then reached a tipping point where something then *broke* inside the person in question. They lost their job, their spouse left them, one of their parents died and then suddenly something snaps and major depression eventuates.

The interesting thing is that some people snap at a certain point, others snap at another point and another group doesn't snap no matter how much stress is heaped on. The only thing people have to go on is there genetic heritage. If you have a depressive parent or one that went through a breakdown of some sort, you clearly have to exercise particular caution in how much stress you allow to permeate your world.

The other problem is that the relationship between stimuli (the stress) and the reaction (a breakdown or depressive episode) is not linear. It is like a dropped coffee cup. If you drop a coffee cup from a small distance above the ground it won't break. Then you raise it up a little higher - it still doesn't break. As you gradually raise the cup up higher, at a certain tipping point if you drop the cup it will shatter. It's not as if each time you drop it, the cup gets a little bit damaged. The stress (hitting the ground) and the relationship to the reaction (the cup breaking) is not linear. At a certain point it goes from "not broken" to "broken". This analogy is helpful because it is easy to visualize but it is not entirely accurate. For this analogy to be accurate in terms of its application to stress, each time you drop the cup you are actually making it a little stronger. The problem is - who knows at what height the cup will suddenly shatter if dropped?

Similarly with chronic stress, in terms of the brain, we see that at a certain point something snaps inside the person and mental illness results. Here is where the cup analogy shines however. If you were to glue the cup back together so all the pieces fit perfectly, now when you drop the cup it shatters from a much lower height. The correlate for this is the unfortunate fact that an episode of major depression makes you susceptible to further episodes.

Major depression is closer to a heart attack in the sense that once it happens, you are dramatically more vulnerable to it happening again. A heart attack doesn't make the heart muscle stronger, whereas the micro-tears on your skeletal muscles that you get from weight training, *do* actually make those muscles stronger. So for most people, occasional bouts of acute stress is like lifting weights. There is a small, survivable shock that makes the *whole* stronger.

However chronic stress is an entire beast altogether. Keep in mind that I have only really addressed one effect of chronic stress (major depression), however as I mentioned earlier there are a raft of other consequences to keep in mind. It would be a mistake to read this and think *Well, I don't have any mental illness in my family and I am able to take all the stress life is able to throw at me.* How about that grandfather that had lifelong hypertension and died early of a heart attack? What about the aunt who developed type 2 diabetes? That breaking point within every person is different. The weakest link in all of us goes first. What is your own weakest link that would be vulnerable to stress? For some people, they develop insomnia. For others, they need to drink alcohol to cope.

When they learn about eustress and distress, many people struggle to discern which is which, as the line between them can become blurred.

Two of the keys are - *control* and a *sense of purpose*.

One of the classic (and cruel - everyone should take a moment to thank animals that suffer for our benefit) experiments done on mice involves subjecting them to electric shocks at random intervals. What researchers find is that if the mice have a degree of control over their environment (such as an ability to quickly escape to a safe zone when the floor becomes electrified), they appear to maintain a relatively unchanged disposition. However, if the shocks come randomly and the mice have no way of escaping, very soon they start manifesting various biomarkers of depression or an anxiety disorder. The difference is control.

A similar mammalian correlate is the difference between an alpha male and a subordinate male in a group of primates. The poor downtrodden monkeys have markedly lower levels of serotonin than the alphas. They are at the mercy of another animal, with no control over their environment.

The human correlate is someone harassed by a despotic boss at work or someone who is dominated by an abusive partner. There is a reason why CEOs often strut around their domain with a pleasant disposition (apart from the fact that that are almost guaranteed to be an extrovert) - their neurobiological status is completely different to the office gopher on the bottom rung of the company ladder.

Likewise, a common trigger for depression in humans is a feeling that their situation is hopeless, beyond their control to ameliorate. Uncontrolled stress is therefore, unsurprisingly, an extremely common trigger for a nervous breakdown (which is really just an outdated expression for major depression) - because it features two potent breakdown triggers - stress and a lack of control.

Let's glance again at the evolutionary forces which underpin so much of our behavior and biology. What happens when an animal is trapped or cornered? Its body is flooded with the biomarkers of its fight or flight system - cortisol, noradrenaline, glucose and various inflammatory substances such as cytokines (in case you need to repair damage from a wound sustained in defending yourself).

Naturally, you can't just magically turn into a CEO, however there are other ways of achieving the same result. As you would imagine, your first task is to work out whether you can indeed just remove yourself (the "flight" in "fight or flight") from whatever it is that possibly makes you feel trapped. Sometimes people have a mental block and believe their situation is inescapable when in fact it is. Often it is possible to leave that abusive partner. Sometimes it is possible to quit your job and change to something less distressing. Here is where the real magic happens. Sometimes just realizing you can escape a situation reduces the stress associated with it. This is because part of the stress is due to the situation itself and part of the stress is due to your perception of it as being inescapable.

However if you can't escape your current situation due to whatever reason, you must then work to reframe it. Let's use weights training as an example. If you are someone who lifts weights at the gym, you are voluntarily subjecting yourself to often intense pain as you push yourself. However, if you were subjected to this same degree of pain each day due to a physical ailment, your stress reaction would be completely different. So the key is not the pain itself but the context under which it arises.

The key is to have a sense of purpose. If you don't even want to escape a situation, it will be significantly less stressful, and even the stress that does remain will not have the same deleterious effects on your health.

An eleven year study of elderly people by the NIH in the US found that those who had a strong sense of purpose lived longer and happier lives than those who didn't. Injecting purpose into a stressful life can be the difference between living past 100 and dying of a sudden heart attack in mid-life. More on sense of purpose later in the book.

Don't accept eustress as unavoidable. Do something about it.

Understand the impact of risky behavior on your life-expectancy

To again use an extreme to illustrate a point, there is no point following every principle mentioned in this book while you spend your weekends base-jumping and driving your car at injudiciously high speeds. If you want to live to 100 and beyond, you need to address not just biological aging, but behavior that exposes your life to risk.

Now for some, the idea of giving up their adrenaline-charged extreme sports sounds like their own personal idea of hell. That's fine. As long as you have a clear idea in your mind of the risks you are exposing yourself to and you are happy with the odds. Depression will also kill you before your time, so clearly you need to do the stuff that makes you happy, dangerous or not.

But remember that risk is cumulative and additive. Let me give the example of driving and skydiving. Skydiving proponents love to defend the safety of the sport (which I admit is much safer than you would imagine). A website I found has arrived at the odds of dying in a parachuting accident as 1 in 100,000 (1 death for every 100,000 jumps), whereas the chance of dying in a motor vehicle accident in any given year is stated as being 1 in 6000.

The first problem with this is where you have multiple jumps each year, as any but the most casual of skydivers would have. Each jump incrementally increases your chances of dying. Each time you repeat a risky activity, you are exposing yourself to additive risk. So if you occasionally speed while driving, it is much less risky than someone who habitually speeds.

The second problem I have with this logic is that it employs a fallacy of logic by comparing driving your car to skydiving. Driving your car is, for many people, an unavoidable part of life. They need to commute to work or to be able to get around and do their shopping. By skydiving (or a similar activity with inherent risk), you are *adding* to the base risk of driving. Unless someone never drives in a car, this comparison is pointless in terms of assessing the relative risk of each activity.

Now I don't mean to pick on skydiving, which actually is a surprisingly safe sport. Many sports have a higher perceived level of risk because the risks are so visible. Skydiving (1 in 100,000 risk) and bungee jumping (1 in 500,000 risk) appear risky because the means of your demise is so readily apparent. In actual fact the riskiest activities are often the ones associated with unlikely means of demise. So before you engage in an activity (either on a regular basis or as a one-off), make sure you have assessed the risks in a logical way.

Remember, the key word is *additive*. Each risk doesn't occur in a vacuum. To give an extreme example, say you ride a motorcycle without a helmet, smoke a pack of cigarettes each day, regularly go base jumping (and yes, I think it would be exceedingly unlikely for someone who smokes a pack a day of cigarettes to go base jumping - this is just for example's sake), drive well over the speed limit, abuse recreational drugs, never exercise and enjoy scuba diving just off Seal Island in South Africa. How likely do you think it would be for you to reach 100? So while the individual risk of an activity is low, the risks increase exponentially each time you repeat the activity and there is also additive risk for each additional other risky activity you engage in.

Here are some of the most common ways to reduce your life expectancy by additive risk -

Use a motorcycle as your main means of transportation. Adding "no helmet" to this puts you in the shallow end of the gene pool.

Smoke cigarettes. Goes without saying right? Here are a couple of damning statistics in case you needed convincing. Lifelong smoking reduces your life expectancy by 25 YEARS. Each packet of cigarettes you smoke, takes 28 minutes off your life. However it is pointless to even mention cigarettes because if you are reading a book on living to 100 and beyond, you are highly unlikely to be a smoker.

Abuse recreational drugs. Each drugs has its own particular risk. For example, heroin is surprisingly non-toxic for the human body (cue hysterical "just say no" people picketing my house). If you were to take oral heroin in controlled dosages, the worst you risk (in terms of damage to the body) is chronic constipation and some relatively benign immune-system issues. The problem with heroin is the dose escalation required to mitigate tolerance and the lack of QC processes wherever the heroin is produced, leading to inconsistent potency and therefore risk of overdose. Not to mention the additive risk of HIV or hepatitis from sharing needles. The contrasts with other drugs like inhalants or methamphetamine (meth), which destroy your body and brain in quick order. If you insist on smoking marijuana, seek out older strains and avoid the newer super-potent strains. Marijuana traditionally had a balanced proportion of *Tetrahydrocannabinol* (which is pro-psychotic) and *cannabidiol* (anti-psychotic). Newer strains have had the cannabidiol bred out, which some researchers believe is the reason why there is such a big problem with marijuana triggering psychotic disorders. If you or your family have any history of schizophrenia, please avoid marijuana altogether.

Drink alcohol in any quantity of 250ml per day. According to the National Cancer Institute, alcohol consumption increases your risk for a range of cancers - particularly cancers of the head or neck, liver, esophagus and breast. If you just read this and you enjoy alcohol, have a quick think about what was the first thought that came into your head when you read this. People are often happy to do anything in books such as these except give up alcohol. Take a moment to ponder what this potentially means regarding your relationship with alcohol. Alcohol is a potent toxin for the body that has just happened to become a social norm. If alcohol was discovered today it would be immediately made illegal. Sorry to sound like a wowser, however it is my responsibility to illuminate all risks. It is then up to you to decide whether you are comfortable with your odds.

These are just a couple of examples. It is up to you to make a clear assessment of the activities you engage in that add to your risk of early death. Perhaps you enjoy jumping into the wild animal enclosures at zoos or something else I have no ability to imagine.

Assess these activities and then make an informed decision as to whether you want to continue. There is nothing wrong with engaging in risky activities that give you a love for life. Just understand the risks involved so you are not taken by surprise when you find yourself walking through a dark tunnel with your dead grandma waiting for you on the other side.

Healthy diet

The problem with dietary recommendations is that the science is constantly evolving. Remember all those years you were told to avoid eggs because they gave you high cholesterol and increased your risk of heart disease? Now eggs are recognized as one of nature's super-foods, with just about every vitamin you need. If I was trapped on a desert island with only one choice of food, eggs would be near the top *(and yes, I realize that I could possibly just order "Asian beef stir fry" or some other complete meal, if I was particularly clever)*.

Similarly, we are in the midst of a major shift in our understanding of nutrition. While there are some nutritionists who are still behind the times and some doctors who disagree, we are seeing the following general trends in nutrition -

- Saturated fat does not "clog your arteries" and is in fact vital for a range of biochemical processes. The villain is in fact trans-fatty acids and polyunsaturated vegetable oils (such as soybean or canola oil). If you are still using margarine instead of (heavenly) butter, you may want to do a little research. If you are still worried about butter, at least switch to spreads made from olive oil.

- Olive oil - speaking of olive oil, it remains the one single fat that everyone agrees is healthy. Some people still believe butter is unhealthy, whereas olive oil remains untouched by controversy.

- Vegetables - and speaking of controversy, vegetables are still the main category of food that everyone agrees is good for you. Particularly leafy greens such as broccoli.

- Whole grains (or any grain-based products) are not particularly healthy. Adding roughage to grain does not miraculously make it healthy if you are eating plenty of fiber-rich vegetables. However there are a few exceptions where there is still healthy debate and ongoing research. For example, rice appears to be a more healthy option than wheat-based products such as bread (Some scientists think this is because rice has a lot of the bad stuff leeched out when it is boiled)

- Legumes - Legumes (such as soy) have vocal supporters and opponents on both sides. Legumes contain some healthy phytochemicals and some not so healthy ones. Do your own research and make up your mind. I tend to think that a few beans here and there don't do me any particular harm. If in doubt, stick to vegetables.

- Avoid quick-digesting carbohydrates such as bread, pasta, rice and potatoes if you want to lose weight.

- Animal protein is good for you and can promote weight loss. This point used to drive opponents of the Atkins weight loss method crazy. They would invent all kinds of explanations why people would lose dramatic amounts of weight eating mainly fat and protein. I have seen similar experiences first hand - people struggling to lose any weight by going "low fat", then switching to Paleo or Atkins-style diets and losing a heap of weight.

- Calories in, calories out - Speaking of losing weight eating animal protein and fat, if someone tries to tell you that weight loss is just a question of "calories in, calories out" tell them that "the 1980s called and they want their weight loss suggestions back". This advice completely ignores the important aspect regarding the hormones that control hunger and what your body does with the energy it consumes. Still skeptical? Tomorrow morning, eat a large serving of white bread. Then, record what time you subsequently become hungry again and the intensity of your hunger. The next morning, eat only animal protein such as meat or egg (try to match the actual calories as closely as possible - you may have to weigh your food). Then measure when you became hungry and how hungry you were. OK, back now? Pretty amazing wasn't it? Eating carbohydrates makes you hungry due to the insulemic response. Eating animal protein keeps you fuller for longer. Remember those morbidly obese people you saw on television who you thought might be just lazy or lacking willpower? It turns out that most of these people have a certain hormonal status (mainly focusing on ghrelin, leptin and insulin) that causes them to rarely feel full and be almost constantly hungry. They are often in a state of perpetual torture. This shows the power of your hormones to control hunger and fat storage. Remember this next time someone tells you that it's all about "calories in, calories out".

- Fruit juice is not healthy - An apple is healthy. A glass of apple juice made from 5-10 apples is not healthy in the slightest. From an evolutionary perspective, your body has no way of processing such a massive blast of sugar as you get from a glass of juice such as apple or orange juice. A glass of juice wreaks havoc on your blood sugar levels and insulin response. Everyone knows that soda is unhealthy, but many people still think that fruit juice is a healthy alternative. It isn't. Stick to water for thirst and if you feel like fruit, eat fruit, not fruit juice.

- Eating a high-fat or high-cholesterol diet gives you heart disease - Tell this to the ethnic groups such as the *Maasai* and the *Inuit* who consume almost entirely animal fat and protein yet experience much less heart disease than westerners. Dietary cholesterol consumption is not only a poor predictor of heart disease but also a poor predictor of serum cholesterol levels! That's right - the majority of your cholesterol level is determined by genetics and liver function, not the amount of cholesterol you consume. One of the greatest scandals in nutrition over the past 50 years has been the lipid hypothesis, which hypothesized that your level of fat consumption determines your risk of heart disease. The frustrating thing was that you are now told to avoid fatty foods because of two dubious events -

  o Ancel Keys' *Seven Countries Study* - this was the first study published that showed a link between fat consumption and heart disease. There's just one problem. There were actually 22 countries' data available and Keys cherry picked the countries that fit his hypothesis. He excluded countries (such as the Netherlands and Norway) where there was a high-fat diet but less heart disease, and countries that consume less fat but have higher heart disease (like Chile).

  o The USDA - Keys' work was picked up by the USDA (whose main function is to promote US grain-based agriculture) and used to promote a grain-based diet. Have a look at the USDA food pyramid -

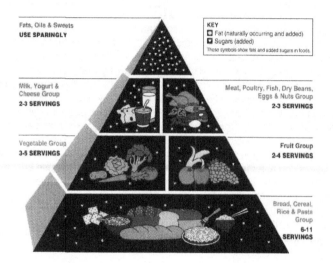

Notice anything odd? Yep - all the foods on the bottom are made from the grains that the USDA promotes. Don't you think it is strange that bread would be on the bottom below vegetables?

- Seafood - Another type of food that is almost free from controversy (similarly to vegetables and olive oil) is seafood - particularly fatty fish that are rich in Omega 3 fatty acids. If you remain nervous about saturated fat and animal protein, a diet focused around seafood and vegetables is a risk-free option. Just avoid fish at the top of the food chain (such as tuna, shark, and swordfish) which can be high in mercury.

- Avoid processed meat - While there is nothing wrong with animal protein, you should avoid processed meat (smoked, cured or in any way processed) which is associated with increased risk of certain cancers such as bowel cancer. Each new study that comes out reinforces this association, including a huge analysis in Europe that looked at more than 400,000 people. No-one knows for sure why this is the case. Some researchers think it is because processed meats (like bacon) are often consumed by people who are not focused on a healthy diet. This is the reason why vegetarian diets are sometimes associated with longer life-expectancy - the average person eating a vegetarian diet is more likely to be concerned about their health and make healthier lifestyle choices. Other researchers think that the problem with processed meats may be their nitrate content. Whatever the reason, there is enough evidence for you to avoid processed meat where possible *(Note - hypocrisy warning - the author wishes to disclose that he has a love affair with bacon and, try as he may, he cannot break the hold that this delicious variety of processed meat has on him)*

So, based on the current science and the information we have, the following foods should form a major part of your diet -

- Leafy green vegetables such as broccoli or Chinese cabbage (*Bok Choy*) - This is as close as you get to the perfect food source

- Seafood - With particular focus on foods rich in omega 3 such as salmon and sardines. Oysters (farmed in areas free of pollution) are a great natural source of zinc.

- Fruit (particularly berries) - Just about every type of fruit has unique selling points. Bananas are packed full of potassium and apples are packed full of a healthy type of fiber called pectin. However the undisputed champions (especially in terms of anti-aging benefits) are berries, which, as previously mentioned, are full of various polyphenols that fight oxidative stress. Plus, berries are relatively lower in fructose.

- If you are going to eat red meat, ensure it is grass-fed (not grain-fed). Grain-fed meat is high in omega 6, whereas grass-fed meat is high in omega 3.

Anti-aging supplements

This tends to be the area that people instinctively get initially attracted to whenever they want to delay the process of aging. There is something seductive and appealing about taking a pill that does all the hard work and you can sit back and reap the rewards. Unfortunately no such pill exists. If it did, everybody would be taking it and you would know its name.

Likewise, no pill is ever going to fully offset poor lifestyle choices. If you spend your life on the couch eating garbage, no pill is going to save you. Anti-aging supplements should be viewed as the last 5%. They are not going to do the heavy-lifting in terms of getting you to 100 and beyond, however they can help prevent certain diseases or aging processes that have the ability to strike you down ahead of time.

Anti-aging supplements can also be quite expensive, so if you can't afford them, don't worry - there are many ways in which you can more than make up for their effects. For example, N-acetylcysteine increases levels of glutathione, but so too does exercise. Curcumin increases levels of BDNF, but again, so too does exercise.

Here are some of the supplements with the strongest research backing in terms of their ability to delay or reverse the biological signs of aging. Note that I have only included substances with either proven efficacy or safety. For example, there are many proponents of hormone injections such as DHEA or human growth hormone, however the safety of this practice is not demonstrated yet. Indeed many categorically believe that these kinds of hormone injects are not safe. Similarly, the anti-rejection drug (it stops organ rejection - it doesn't stop someone denying your entreaties for affection) *sirolimus* (*rapamycin*) has shown a promising ability to increase the life-span of mice, however this is also just at the research stage.

Resveratrol - As mentioned earlier, exhibits the ability to increase longevity in mice by mimicking the effects of caloric restriction. However significant questions still remain regarding its bioavailability and ability to actually increase longevity *in vivo*.

CoQ10 - Promotes mitochondrial function and cardiac health.

Curcumin - Reduces inflammation, protects against certain types of cancer and increases levels of BDNF in the brain

N-acetylcysteine - A powerful agent for increasing levels of glutathione

Milk thistle - A powerful liver herb that also increases levels of glutathione

Omega 3 (fish oil and/or krill oil) - A virtually compulsory supplement that supports brain and heart health along with reducing levels of systemic inflammation

Alpha lipoic acid - Another powerful supplement for increasing glutathione

However in addition to those option, there is an exciting "new kid on the block" (in terms of newness, not in terms of resemblance to an 80s teen pop group) – *nicotinamide mononucleotide* (or NMN for those like me who are too lazy to type it out over and over).

NMN has recently begun receiving mainstream attention due to the strong research emerging supporting potent anti-aging effects. Researchers involved in the Australian study have expressed optimism that NMN could treat some of the most common aspects of aging including cancer, type 2 diabetes and inflammatory conditions.

So, how does this miracle substance work? Once again it turns out that those pesky mitochondria are responsible for many of the problems we associate with aging. NMN functions as a precursor to NAD (*nicotinamide adenine dinucleotide*), which is a vital signaling molecule used by mitochondria that declines as we age. Researchers have found that by boosting NAD through NMN, they are able to trigger dramatic anti-aging effects in mice. What is most interesting is that NMN appears to trigger a biological anti-aging effect that mimics the benefits of caloric restriction and exercise. I can tell you, the minute they release a pill that mimics caloric restriction but doesn't have the "caloric restriction" requirement, I will be first in the queue.

Also, NMN appears to also function as a "super resveratrol", boosting a much wider range of sirtuins implicated in the anti-aging process.

The downside? As this is still pre-clinical trial and strictly still only a research chemical, NMN will currently cost you around $40,000 per month (or around $1000 per gram). If you are wealthy enough to pay $40,000 per month for NMN, you are probably also wealthy enough to pay the guy that told you about NMN $40,000. If this describes you, just drop me an email and I can give you my bank details or arrange for a cash pickup. Sorry I don't accept checks at this stage, but could be swayed with a sweetener.

In addition to NMN there is a huge range of unreleased, experimental and pre-clinical trial substances which you can often gain access to if you know where to look. If you are keen to go down this path and don't feel like a guinea pig, probably the best place to start is the Longecity forum. As you will note, there are a range of sub forums. I tend to spend most of my time on the Brain Health forum (under a secret alias!). Quite often, an enterprising forum member will arrange a "group buy", where forum members can pool demand to buy a commercial quantity of a particular obscure anti-aging or nootropic drug or supplement.

Some potential supplements and drugs which are not publicly available could be – NSI-189, D-Deprenyl, Cerebrolysin, GHK tripeptide, nicotinamide riboside (see earlier section on NAD+), GDF11 and many more.

Caloric restriction

Possibly the most potent way to slow down biological aging is unfortunately also the least palatable for most people - myself included. Studies have consistently showed that by dramatically reducing the number of calories a mouse or a human consumes, a raft of biological changes occur which leads to slow aging.

However my view would probably be shared by most people - any life where I can't eat the things I love is not worth living. I would probably last a month or so on caloric restriction before I would die tragically in a self-inflicted, shotgun-related mishap.

According to Eric Ravussin, a human health and performance researcher at the Pennington Biomedical Research Center in Louisiana, 15% less calories from age 25 could bestow upon you a grand total of 4 and a half years extra longevity. *No thanks.*

Even if you decide that you can handle the idea of lifelong caloric restriction, the majority of people soon give up, tired of feeling hungry all the time. It's no way to live.

A more palatable but less potent way of mimicking the effects of caloric restriction would be via resveratrol supplementation, which appears to work via similar mechanisms, as mentioned earlier in this book.

But perhaps a better option for those that can handle it would be to try one of the various forms of intermittent fasting, which involves periods of low or no calories interspersed with normal eating.

Intermittent fasting has compelling research results to back it up as a means to extend life-span. It appears to -

1. Reduce oxidative damage - It is theorized that when you are fasting and your body is not dedicating its internal resources to the process of digestion, it is able to dedicate those resources to repair work.

2. Increase insulin sensitivity - This leads to less incidence of type 2 diabetes and other problems caused by high blood sugar

3. Improved mitochondrial function

In general, intermittent fasting appears to act via the same mechanism I mentioned in the section on stress - *hormesis*. It is a kind of small, survivable shock to the organism that increases its overall robustness and resistance to disease.

More specifically, the most obvious mechanism for the beneficial effects of intermittent fasting appears to be the effects on IGF-1 (*insulin-like growth factor 1*). This kind of fasting decreases the expression of IGF-1 (which is called "insulin-like" because it has a similar molecular structure to insulin), a hormone that is central to the anabolic growth of cells. Deficiencies in either IGF-1 or human growth hormone (which is largely controlled by IGF-1) result in stunted growth problems. According to Professor Valter Longo of the

University of Southern California, by decreasing the expression of IGF-1, there is a temporary switch from a growth focus to a repair focus, leading to less damage accumulating over the longer term.

So how important is IGF-1 to longevity? Mice bred to have very low levels of IGF-1 expression live for 40% longer than their standard counterparts. What about humans with low levels of IGF-1 expression? That would be the people with the rare condition *Laron syndrome*, who have unusually low levels of IGF-1 expression. As you would expect, they are much smaller than the average person as they lack the growth hormone mediated anabolic effects we typically have. However, slightly more surprising is the fact that sufferers of Laron syndrome experience much lower rates of diabetes and cancer. Clearly, IGF-1 is a powerful mediator of longevity and our most powerful means to achieve reduced IGF-1 expression at the moment is intermittent fasting.

The other attractive benefit of intermittent fasting for longevity, is that it can lead to often dramatic weight loss. This flies in the face of previously accepted wisdom that recommended regular small meals as the best way to lose weight because this "stokes the fires of your metabolism". The tide of opinion is gradually turning against this line of thinking. This is due partly to the fact that most people's experience is that intermittent fasting sheds weight more effectively, but also due to what we are now learning about the longevity-enhancing effects of periods of time spent without eating food.

How you implement intermittent fasting is largely up to you, as the key appears to be the calories cut rather than any particular way in which each block of eating and fasting is constructed. You can either try - *alternate day fasting* (ADF) which involves one day of normal eating followed by a day of fasting, or the *5:2 diet*, which involves two ultra-low calorie days (they must not be on consecutive days) and five days of normal eating.

Personally I have tried the 5:2 diet and while I found it easier than I expected, it was not something I felt I could maintain for any meaningful period of time. If you want to try this, experiment with what works for you. The key is to find the option that requires the least amount of willpower, as this will be the option with the highest chances of success for you personally.

Meantime, from my perspective, a much more palatable way of achieving similar anti-aging effects to CR is via substances which activate or modulate sirtuin activity, such as nicotinamide riboside.

Get good quality sleep

The connection between stress, elevated cortisol levels and a host of negative health consequences is reasonably well known. What is less widely known is that regularly sleeping less than six hours per night has the exact same effects on the body as chronic stress, including increased cortisol, systemic inflammation and a weakened immune system.

The problem is that this situation applies to more than 30% of all Americans. I don't have any data on the rest of the western world, however I would hazard a guess that the rate is roughly similar when averaged out.

The biggest study into the link between sleep duration and mortality found that sleeping less than six hours per night was associated with a 12% increase in risk of death. Where it gets really interesting is when we see that sleeping more than nine hours per night is associated with a 30% increase in risk of death!

However we need to remember than correlation doesn't equal causation. For example, poor health can cause increased sleep duration in some cases, which would account for the increased risk of death. Similarly, a painful or disabling health condition could be impacting sleep, leading to less time spent asleep.

What we do know however, is that deliberately depriving an animal of sleep can lead to its swift demise. Other studies where subjects are allowed to sleep but are woken as soon as they enter deep (slow wave) sleep also show interesting results. Even though these subjects are getting some of the stages of sleep, without slow wave sleep they literally fall apart, with severe fatigue and even widespread pain that mimics fibromyalgia (*As an aside, the fact that depriving a healthy subject of slow wave sleep appears to cause temporary fibromyalgia, this points to a possible mechanism, among many others, behind this disorder*)

Conservatively however, if we accept these numbers on face value, it would be safe to assume that somewhere between six and nine hours is the "sweet spot" in terms of sleep duration and longevity.

If we look at all the negative health consequences of chronic sleep deprivation, we see an eerie correlation with stress. Sleep deprivation appears to act as a kind of stressor, leading to all the same problems. The main difference is that sleep deprivation manages to achieve all the nasty stuff that stress does, but in a fraction of the time. While the effects of chronic stress slowly build over time, just a few nights of little or no sleep can break even the most durable mind. It's no coincidence that sleep deprivation is an effective torture technique.

There is a kind of "chicken and the egg" relationship between sleep and mental illness. Sleep deprivation is a strong trigger for mental illness and mental illness itself leads to sleep disorders (early morning awakenings, insomnia etc.). Considering that it is during slow wave sleep when your neurotransmitters and hormones (particularly growth hormone) undergo their main process of replenishment, getting insufficient sleep is a recipe for disaster.

What is less clear is the importance of REM (rapid eye movement) sleep on longevity, as the function of REM sleep is still not proven. What we do know, however, is that major depression is associated with increased levels of REM sleep and less slow wave sleep. As most SSRI antidepressants suppress REM sleep, some have hypothesized that suppressing REM sleep (if you have too much of it due to depression) is one of the keys to treating mood disorders. Interestingly, if you artificially prevent a depressed person from experiencing REM sleep by depriving them of sleep, their mood improves dramatically. Unfortunately, this effect only lasts until they next go to sleep - when they wake up again, their depression will remain. Complete sleep deprivation is not a particularly compliance-friendly treatment in any case.

Sleep deprivation not only leads to immediate health consequences, it also causes downstream problems. For example, a lack of sleep leads to disturbances in the appetite-related hormones ghrelin and leptin. This then leads to weight gain, causing a new constellation of problems.

But perhaps the most instantaneous of possible consequences is regarding accidents caused by sleep deprivation. These accidents can go from car accidents caused by fatigue, to the space shuttle *Challenger* disaster, which is believed to have been precipitated indirectly by sleep deprivation.

You need to prioritize sleep ahead of virtually all else, save for drinking water. Nothing will cause things to unravel quicker than sleep deprivation. Unfortunately, for many, sleep comes last in the queue - they will prioritize everything else (work, social engagements, television etc.) ahead of sleep and then sleep duration is just made up of whatever is left, time-wise.

However, sleep is not just a function of duration. Sleep quality must also be preserved and enhanced. If you drink a bottle of wine and fall into a coma for 8 hours, your sleep quality will look completely different to a typical sleep EEG (*electroencephalogram*). Alcohol is poison for sleep quality as it keeps you in the lighter stages of sleep all night. Just another reason why being an alcoholic is up there with cigarette smoking in terms of toxicity to the body and early mortality.

In terms of improving sleep quality, some keys are -

- Avoid alcohol and caffeinated beverages in the evening. Alcohol prevents you from entering into deep sleep and caffeine messes with adenosine levels. Adenosine levels gradually increase during the day and eventually signal your body to sleep at night. Caffeine inhibits this process, reducing sleep quality and often causing insomnia in susceptible individuals.

- Avoid eating too much at night. Sleep quality while digesting a heavy meal is poor.

- Practice relaxation techniques such as meditation or progressive muscle relaxation in the evening.

- Try a warm bath before bed. This has been shown to increase levels of slow wave sleep by accentuating the drop in body temperature that accompanies sleep. Because your body has to cool you down by a greater degree after a bath (as your core temperature is higher), you sleep more deeply. Scientists are still unsure why this actually works, but it does.

If you want further motivation, perhaps clinical trial results may help. Multiple studies have shown that insomniacs have significantly greater levels of oxidative stress than healthy controls (those without insomnia). For example, Gulec et al stated *"Our results show that the patients with primary insomnia had significantly lower GSH-Px activity and higher MDA levels compared with the controls"* and therefore *"These results may indicate the important role of sleep in attenuating oxidative stress"*. Whether you look at it from the perspective of cortisol or oxidative stress, not getting sufficient sleep clearly accelerates the aging process.

So what about sleeping tablets?

While many people tend to get a bit hysterical over sleeping tablets (primarily due to perceived addiction risk), I think you have to get pragmatic sometimes. If it's a choice between chronic insomnia and taking a pill, I will take a pill every time. But there are a few caveats and key points.

Sleeping tablets should be a measure of last resort or used for occasional insomnia - It's no use drinking beer and coffee every night or doing your work presentations on your laptop in bed and wondering why you can't sleep. Before you resort to sleeping tablets, make sure your house is in order in terms of sleep hygiene.

The main reasons why doctors exercise caution regarding sleeping tablets is that (in general - there are some exceptions I will get to in a moment) they give you poor quality sleep and they do carry some addiction risk.

If you visit your doctor complaining of insomnia, depending on the doctor and what country you are in, you will most likely be prescribed either a benzodiazepine (such as temazepam, diazepam or alprazolam) or one of the newer, related "z-drugs" such as zolpidem (*Ambien, Stillnox*), zaleplon (*Sonata*) or eszopiclone (*Lunesta*). There are a range of problems with benzodiazepines which mean that they are being prescribed less and less for sleep problems (they are however, extremely helpful for severe anxiety and panic disorders). They rob you of vital slow wave sleep, which can be deleterious over long periods of time. They also carry the risk of addiction or physical dependence if used at high doses for extended periods. While the risk of addiction to benzodiazepines is often overstated, you don't want to try your luck. Poly-drug users often mention that withdrawing from benzodiazepines like alprazolam (*Xanax*) or clonazepam (*Klonopin*) is worse than heroin. In fact, along with alcohol withdrawal, benzodiazepine withdrawal is one of the only other drugs where the withdrawal process can be life threatening if done incorrectly.

The beauty of z-drugs is that, while they also carry the risk of dependence, they don't wreck your sleep architecture to the same degree.

If you have severe, life-long insomnia however, the longevity-promoting effects of getting sleep will far outweigh any consequences of taking sleeping tablets for extended periods of time. However if you require indefinite assistance to help you sleep, it is better to look at options which are indicated for long term use and which don't ruin your sleep quality. Some potential options include -

Mirtazapine (*Remeron, Avanza, Zispin*) - This is an antidepressant that essentially functions as a super-potent sedating antihistamine with relatively weak antidepressant and anti-anxiety effects. If your sleep problems are caused by underlying issues with depression, this can be a good option. Mirtazapine actually improves sleep quality, in contrast to the benzodiazepines. The major downside is weight gain, which has its own health issues. Mirtazapine users have said that being on the drug is like having the perpetual "munchies".

Promethazine (*Phenergan*) or **diphenhydramine** (*Benadryl*) - These are two older sedating antihistamines which you can get OTC (over the counter) in most countries. Like mirtazapine and other antihistamines, usually improve sleep quality. Some people however react badly to antihistamines and feel groggy the next day. The best part about antihistamines is that they have a long history of safe use. You are unlikely to suddenly grow an extra leg after using them.

Pregabalin (*Lyrica*) or **gabapentin** (*Neurontin*) - These were developed as anticonvulsants but are now used mainly for neuropathic pain (such as fibromyalgia or post-herpetic neuralgia) and anxiety disorders. Both of these drugs improve sleep quality dramatically. They appear to do this by reducing levels of excitatory neurotransmitters such as glutamate, noradrenaline (norepinephrine) and substance P. People tend to either love them or hate them, with many stopping treatment soon after beginning due to intolerable side-effects. Like mirtazapine, the other main problem is weight gain.

There are some other options as well, however for one reason or another, they are not viable. There are the older tricyclic antidepressants (such as amitriptyline), which improve sleep quality at the expense of cardiac function and anticholinergic problems. There is also sodium oxybate (*Xyrem*), which is one of the most potent drugs available for increasing slow wave sleep. The main problem is that sodium oxybate is another name for *GHB*, an illegal street drug. If you are able to successfully convince your doctor to prescribe Xyrem for you, send me their details and I will go and get some from them myself!

Remember though, that there is no such thing as a free lunch. Any extended pharmaceutical use will have consequences, no matter how benign. You just need to weigh up the consequences of this versus long term insomnia, which has deleterious effects on the brain that far outweighs even the most toxic of sleeping tablets (unless perhaps if you need to start sniffing glue to get some shut-eye).

However you need to realize that insomnia rarely occurs in a vacuum. It is generally a symptom of something else, either behavioral (you read work emails in bed just before you are about to go to sleep or something similarly non-conducive to sleep) or neurochemical (underlying depression or anxiety). Occasionally someone has some innate biological problem getting to sleep, however I believe that these people are exceedingly rare. So the best course of action generally is to address whatever is causing your insomnia, use sleeping tablets as a short term solution to get you through, and if nothing works, investigate longer-term options for pharmacological assistance.

Maintain a healthy immune system

We only have to look at HIV AIDS to see what happens when your immune system becomes compromised. However, did you know that the immune system is also responsible for controlling many types of cancer? When a cell "goes rogue" and switches off its own apoptosis (programmed cell death), it is the immune system that identifies and neutralizes the threat before it can develop into cancer.

Imagine your immune system is like a group of soldiers defending a city (your body). Whenever they find an external invader (like a bacteria or virus), they are easily identified and taken care of. However cancer cells are a little trickier. Cancer cells are like a rogue traitorous soldier who has decided to join the enemy. Because they are wearing the uniform of the "home team", they are not as easy to identify. Therefore, occasionally something slips through the defenses and can turn into a cancer.

However a key determinant of how good your immune system "soldiers" are at keeping the cancer cells at bay is overall immune function. If you have compromised immune function or a lifestyle that triggers too many cells to "go rogue", you are increasing your chances of developing cancer.

And immune function is not just related to cancer. A compromised immune system is one of the major problems associated with old age. Young, healthy subjects with full-strength immune systems don't develop pneumonia regularly. A weakened immune system is one of the fundamental hallmarks of the aging process. One of the main reasons for this is the gradual decline in your body's ability to manufacture new *T lymphocytes* (T-cells) and B *lymphocytes* (B-cells) which make up part of your front line defense.

Therefore, quite a bit of research has been directed at either reversing the atrophy of your thymus (the organ that produces T-cells – hence the "T") or reactivating white blood cells. Until recently, it was thought that white blood cells became inactive due to telomere shortening. However recent research has indicated that may not be the case and that it may be possible to re-activate the white blood cells. One of the researchers in this particular study likened it to bring football players out of retirement and back into the game.

While specific therapies emerging out of this research are some time off, we are fortunate in the meantime that we already have a variety of ways to support and regenerate immune system function. For example, if we stay on the subject of the thymus, dietary zinc supplements have been showed to have a beneficial effect on thymus size and function. A 2009 study by Wong et al found *"...that in mice, zinc supplementation can reverse some age-related thymic defects and may be of considerable benefit in improving immune function and overall health in elderly populations".*

In terms of supplementation, the following all have good, solid research backing –

Curcumin – Yes, curcumin again. Is there anything it can't do?

Garlic – There is some evidence that garlic possesses some immune-boosting effects.

Due to the sulfur content, you should already be eating a diet rich in garlic anyway

Astragalus – This has a long history of use in Chinese medicine as an immune system herb. Some interesting preliminary research suggests that astragalus may increase telomerase activity. A proprietary extract of astragalus appears to reduce the extent to which T-cells become senescent and inactive.

Olive leaf extract – As well as acting as an anti-microbial (it fights bacteria, viruses and fungi), olive leaf extract also appears to stimulate phagocytosis, which is where your *macrophagocytes* (another one of your immune system's army of soldiers) attack and engulf a pathogen.

This is just a few of the various supplements and herbs which may have immune-boosting effects. There are a range of other options also, including – Echinacea, goldenseal and vitamin C.

Unfortunately however, there are no supplements that could be considered to have proven and reproducible effects on the immune system. For example, some studies have shown echinacea to be of benefit, whereas others did not.

Fortunately however, we have a much more powerful way of modulating the immune system to prevent age-related decline. Unfortunately, however, I am going to sound like a broken record because the most powerful way to maintain a healthy, functioning immune system is to manage and avoid chronic stress.

Ever noticed how, during a period of intense stress you suddenly come down with a cold? It's no co-incidence. Scientists have known for a long time now that there is a strong connection between stress levels and your immune system. Your immune system and your sympathetic nervous system (your fight or flight system that prepares you for action) have a rich network of various type of connections. For example, many of the cells that your immune system uses to fight pathogens, such as lymphocytes, have special receptors for various substances produced during periods of stress, such as noradrenaline and endorphins. Research has consistently found that stress reduces the activity of natural killer cells and suppresses the proliferation of lymphocytes.

Also, consistent with what I mentioned in the section on stress, it appears clear that time-limited, acute stress (such as the stress before an exam) enhances immune response, while chronic stress (such as an abusive relationship or a stressful job) suppresses immune response.

If you can prevent or eliminate chronic stress, you are able to ameliorate much of the age-related decline in immune response. This by no means confers a 100 year old the immune system of a teenager. There are still age-related declines in immune function that will occur in everybody. However, I am hopeful that one of the current research projects throws up a novel agent that is able to identify and mitigate the worst of our age-related decline in immune function.

Another factor which many believe to be central to immune system status is vitamin D levels. Yes, vitamin D. Again. There is a strong correlation between vitamin D levels and immune function. Some scientists believe this may be one of the factors as to why we get colds and flu more often in the winter time when we naturally get less sun exposure. So ensure that you get at least 20 minutes per day of sun exposure and take vitamin D supplements (with vitamin K as well).

Sensible use of medication where appropriate

There is an old saying that says the only difference between a poison and a medicine is the dose. 1 tablet (500mg) of acetaminophen (paracetamol) will relieve pain and reduce a fever. Take twenty of them and you risk liver failure and death.

People can sometimes become too fundamental and dogmatic regarding pharmaceuticals. Yes, pharmaceuticals are largely developed by "Big Pharma" with profit in mind, but the end result is that they often reduce suffering in the world.

There is no *one size fits all* blanket statement that one can make regarding pharmaceuticals. The key question you need to ask yourself is - *Am I reducing my life expectancy by taking this drug or not taking this drug?* Sure, many drugs can have negative effects on the body (particularly the liver and brain), but these effects need to be weighed up against the alternative.

Here are some general guidelines for certain types of medications -

Statins

Statins are not inherently "evil" as some people make them out to be. They have just been misused by the marketing department of pharmaceutical companies. If you have already had a heart attack, been diagnosed with a form of heart disease or suffer from hypercholesterolemia (unhealthily high natural cholesterol levels), statins have been proven to save lives. The problem comes with the marketing. Pharmaceutical companies cleverly realized that if they could get the definition of "high cholesterol" and "at risk person" widened, they could dramatically increase the market size for statins. What has happened since has been one of the most deviously brilliant marketing and lobbying campaigns in the history of medicine. So now we have a situation where someone can visit the doctor with slightly elevated cholesterol and be put on statins. Statins have demonstrated no statistically significant ability to reduce the risk of heart disease in healthy people. However, if you are one of the at risk groups mentioned above, statins can be a lifesaver and a compulsory medicine. Don't form a dogmatic view against statins that prevents you from getting adequate care. Take time to educate yourself on the risk/benefit ratio. You need to weigh up the potential benefit of preventing a heart attack with the increased risk of diabetes, dementia or muscle problems that some researchers have linked to statins. As an interesting aside, researchers are now saying that the reason why statins can be beneficial for some is that they act as anti-inflammatories. If this is the case, personally, I would stick to omega 3, vitamin D and curcumin supplements to achieve the same result but without the side-effects.

If you do decide to take statins, please ensure you also take CoQ10 at the same time and get adequate vitamin D from the sun and also vitamin D supplements.

SSRI antidepressants

Another area where people can get infuriatingly dogmatic. At one end of the spectrum you have people who believe that antidepressants are evil and cause brain damage. At the other end you have those who believe that depression can be explained simply in terms of monoamine neurotransmitters such as serotonin. As with anything, the truth lies somewhere in the middle.

So, let me cut through the spin to lay down some simple facts -

Antidepressants work for most people to treat symptoms of depression and/or anxiety. If in doubt, don't generate your opinion based on what you read on internet forums. Internet forums on depression feature something called selection bias, which means they are not an accurate reflection of reality. The people who are on depression forums complaining that their antidepressants don't work give a skewed picture of reality. This is because if you take antidepressants and get better, you won't spend your time on the internet talking about your experience. You will have moved on.

Antidepressants don't cause brain damage - If anything, they have been proven to do the opposite. SSRI (selective serotonin reuptake inhibitors such as *Prozac, Zoloft* and *Lexapro*) therapy is associate with areas of the brain (primarily the hippocampus) re-growing, after depression has initially caused atrophy. SSRIs increased levels of BDNF, your brain's important "fertilizer".

Antidepressants don't "cure" depression. Firstly, there is no such thing as *curing* depression, only achieving *remission*. Secondly, treating depression should be done holistically, looking at - cognition, behavior, diet and other factors. Sitting back and waiting for a pill to do all the hard work is not only less effective, but means that when you go off your drugs, you are more likely to become depressed again. Depression is (in most cases) caused by something. You have to fix whatever that *something* is. A pill doesn't do that.

Depression is not "caused" by low serotonin - Depression is a hugely complex beast that still eludes a clean and simple explanation. So many different biological and psychological systems are involved that, to reduce everything down to serotonin is misguided. We don't even clearly know whether low serotonin causes depression or depression causes low serotonin. Likewise, while we know that SSRIs work, many scientists believe they work for reasons completely independent of serotonin. For example, there is a drug called tianeptine *(Stablon)*, which acts as a selective serotonin reuptake enhancer and works as an effective antidepressant. That's right - it does the exact opposite thing in your brain to SSRIs (which inhibit the reuptake of serotonin), yet treats depression. The brain is infinitely more complex than we can imagine.

Depression can be deadly. Depending on the figures you use, there are between 30,000 and 50,000 suicide deaths each year in the US alone. To withhold appropriate treatment because of dogmatic opposition or worries about the health consequences of SSRIs is insane. SSRIs have no proven link with lowered life expectancy apart from the small number of people who commit suicide shortly after beginning treatment.

However, I should also point out, that for mild to moderate cases of depression, drugs don't perform any better than placebo. Interestingly, the most effective treatment for mild to moderate depression is also one of the potent anti-agers mentioned earlier - cardiovascular exercise. In Jump Start - An introduction to the science of exercise therapy for anxiety & depression, Benjamin Kramer says *"Study after study has clearly shown that cardiovascular exercise and/or weight training works just as well as antidepressant medication, but with one key advantage - Those subjects who treat their anxiety and depression with exercise tend to stay well, whereas those who treat their depression with medication have a significantly higher relapse rate"*.

Prescription stimulants for ADHD

If there was ever a candidate for the most controversial area of modern psychopharmacology, it would be the use of stimulants (such as methylphenidate and amphetamine-related drugs) to treat ADD and ADHD.

Firstly, yes, these stimulants are, in some ways, toxic for the brain. You would never take these drugs to achieve lasting, positive change in the brain.

Secondly, yes, they probably are over-prescribed - used in milder cases where behavioral intervention would be more appropriate.

However, if you have ever had any experience with the use of these drugs to treat more severe cases of ADHD, you would know that they are usually spectacularly successful. They can (in less than an hour) cause the most dramatic improvements in functioning imaginable. They can take a child, who is being both self-destructive and destructive to those around them, and create a normal, placid, fully-functioning child. The changes that can occur are sometimes nothing short of amazing. Families who have gotten their life back thanks to these medications understandably get angry when they read an academic or journalist claim that these drugs aren't helpful or that ADHD doesn't even exist.

Some believe that ADHD itself is an invented illness. Sure, this may be the case. However in my opinion, more weight must be given to the reduction in suffering of these kids than to any problems with the theory behind ADHD.

If you or your children are unable to function or lead a normal life due to the range of symptoms we call "ADHD" or "ADD", the negative effects on longevity of taking these drugs would be far outweighed by the longevity-shortening effects of not seeking appropriate pharmacological help.

Vaccines

To be honest, I find it amazing that I even have to mention vaccines. There is a special place in hell reserved for parents who refuse to vaccinate their child. The most frustrating part is that the only reason there are people suspicious of vaccines is because of a study in the UK that was later proven to be fraudulent. This fraudulent research paper garnered significant media attention and led to an immediate drop in vaccinations by panicked parents because it appeared to show that vaccines cause autism. This was predictably followed by an increase in the number of reported cases of measles and mumps.

However, here is where things get truly bizarre. Despite the fact that this study was universally proven to be fraudulent (by all but the most whacko of conspiracy theorists), the idea that vaccines cause autism remained in the minds of certain parents. This is the equivalent of someone telling you there is a bogeyman in your closet, then admitting they were only joking, yet you continue to believe the bogeyman is there.

Get your child vaccinated. End of story. According to the World Health Organization (WHO), 2.5 million deaths are prevented each year by vaccines.

Fortunately in the last couple of years, the label "anti-vaxxer" has become pejorative as the public has gradually realized the impacts on herd immunity caused by a small minority of "concerned parents". Whilst hardcore anti-vaxxers are unlikely to ever see the light, this should have the effect of convincing the fence-sitters through a combination of peer pressure and awareness campaigns.

Yes, Big Pharma is out to get your money and will often push the boundaries of what is ethical (statins being case in point). However this is no grounds for denying yourself or your children access to what can often be life-saving medicines.

Don't be swayed by websites and their vague, unscientific claims regarding "toxins" in vaccines. Get vaccinated.

There are countless other medications and conditions that may need medicating - this is just a few of the main ones. Remember, everyone is different. For someone with ADHD, taking a stimulant medication can be longevity enhancing (because benefits across multiple parts of their life can outweigh the negative consequences of stimulants). For someone without ADHD, these drugs are just toxic stimulants.

If you have a health condition, get appropriate treatment (whether with drugs or otherwise). If not, stay away from unnecessary pharmaceuticals.

General tips for getting you to 100 and beyond

Here are some more tips that don't fit into any of the other categories -

Get regular check-ups

This is one that many people are guilty of - they are so scared of the doctor's office that they avoid getting regular check-ups. Both my mother and grandmother died of problems that may have been treatable if they had sought help earlier. My mother knew something was wrong for a year before she was finally coerced into getting help. Remember this key fact - most cancers are curable if caught early. Cancer is not the death sentence it once was. However, once cancer has metastasized (spread) it becomes infinitely more difficult to treat, so you need to keep on top of things. If your doctor can identify and treat various problems early, your chances of beating them increase exponentially.

Order various tests

There are a range of tests that can be extremely helpful in illuminating existing or potential illnesses. The problem is that, unless your doctor has a specific concern, they won't order a test unless requested to.

The *c-reactive protein* (CRP) test is a great example. This test is used to detect inflammation in the body and is traditionally used to screen for heart disease where there is inflammation of the arteries suspected. A study that measured the CRP levels of 1100 men found that those with elevated CRP has triple the risk of heart disease and double the risk of stroke compared to those with normal or low levels. The CRP test is fantastic for identifying the very beginnings of heart disease, allowing you to put in place measures to prevent a possible heart attack from full-blown heart disease.

However there is also an association with elevated CRP and certain cancers. If you acknowledge that inflammation is one of the central factors in aging, then an accurate means to measure it is vital. When you ask for this test, make sure you ask for it in terms of your concern regarding heart disease.

At the same time, if you ask for a lipid panel to measure cholesterol, the key value to focus on is your triglycerides. Elevated triglycerides, which are associated with excess carbohydrate consumption, are increasingly being viewed as the best predictor of heart disease. While on the subject of lipid panel, try to get a particle-size test done. This measures the particle size of the lipoproteins because some particle sizes are benign, whereas others are harmful.

Some other tests to ask for including - vitamin D status, liver function, comprehensive metabolic panel, thyroid-stimulating hormone, complete blood cell count, fibrinogen, hemoglobin a1c, DHEA.

Some of these will be available and some you may need to visit a specialist laboratory.

Quantified self

Closely linked to the above topic of medical tests is the growing movement called quantified self. What this entails is measuring all aspects of your life empirically to enable to you to make positive changes or identify potential problems.

Probably the aspect of quantified self that you would be most familiar is pedometers that track the number of steps you take each day. This embodies one of the key concepts of quantified self - if you can measure something, you can improve it.

I own a *FitBit* tracker which I wear wherever I go. It tracks the number of steps, the distance, how many flights of stairs, calories burned and sleep quality. It tells me when I have been cooped up in my room writing for too long. I try to make it to 10,000 steps each day so when I find myself falling short, I go for a walk just to get to my target. This one little device has dramatically increased my activity levels. Unless I am in a skyscraper, I rarely ever take elevators any more, as I want to beat my record for most number of flights I have walked up in one day (currently 60 flights). I am a fan of FitBit but there are many different options so shop around if necessary.

Quantified self doesn't just refer to pedometers. It can refer to measuring various aspects of your body (waist size, weight etc.) and tracking the effects of certain activities. The central concept is that you can't improve what you can't measure. People can go years without weighing themselves or measuring their waistline then one day they hop on the scales and see a horrific number staring back at them. If you regularly track things like this, you have more opportunity to nip problems in the bud. Just don't go overboard. Remember, weight fluctuates wildly over a 24 or eve 48 hour period so don't keep weighing yourself each day. Once a week is enough - and make sure it's done at the same time each day.

Similarly, with a good quality blood pressure machine, if you take regular readings you will be able to identify and deal with any hypertension-related problems. Remember, hypertension (high blood pressure) is a silent killer. A good quality blood pressure machine could be the difference between life and death – literally.

Meditate regularly

Meditation has a range of longevity-enhancing effects, but the key benefit is secondary. Meditation is one of the best ways to combat chronic stress, which, as we know from earlier, is a huge driver of early death. Meditation leads to a range of physiological effects that reduce levels of stress, anxiety and depression.

Meditation is such a powerful anti-stress technique, that a whole new branch of psychotherapy, called *mindfulness-based stress reduction* (MBSR) has emerged as a popular way to fight stress and mood disorders. A 2003 meta-analysis found the MBSR was helpful not just for these obvious stress-related problems, but also for other conditions such as fibromyalgia, heart disease and certain other pain-related conditions.

Recent research into the effects of meditation on the brain, using fMRI and similar brain-scanning techniques, has thrown up some amazing results. One of the pioneers of this has been Professor Richard Davidson, director of the Laboratory for Affective

Neuroscience at the University of Wisconsin, who has worked with the Dalai Lama to measure the brains of long term meditators. Among other things, Professor Davidson found that Tibetan lamas who had brains that were unlike any he had previously measured. When you think happy thoughts, certain parts of your brain (such as the left prefrontal cortex) light up. When you think negative or fearful thoughts, other parts light up (such as the right prefrontal cortex and the amygdala). Professor Davidson found a correlation between the number of hours someone meditates and the level of, what could subjectively be called "happiness".

The good news is that, while beginner meditators didn't have the extreme level of positive emotion in their brain after meditating, there were definite positive changes. These benefits of meditation slowly accrue over the long term.

Meditation also has direct effects on cellular aging. In particular, long term meditation is associated with higher levels of the important hormone DHEA, which usually decreases gradually as you age. Lower levels of DHEA (which is sometimes referred to as the "youth hormone") have been implicated in a range of conditions such as heart disease, diabetes and cancer. DHEA is considered so important, that many people have experimented with controversial DHEA supplementation. DHEA supplements are available in the US, but are still banned in most countries. My own personal philosophy is that I avoid any of these direct hormonal treatments such as DHEA or human growth hormone, as the research isn't yet conclusive regarding the risk/benefit ratio. The only hormone I supplement with is vitamin D (yes, it's a hormone and not actually a vitamin – fun fact!).

While meditation is now a mainstream, proven technique for stress reduction, there is still a huge amount of ignorance that prevents people from benefiting. Here are a couple of the main ones -

Meditation is against my religion - When it is boiled down to its purest essence, meditation is just a process of calming the mind and looking clearly at your own thought processes. Meditation (when used in a clinical setting) has become largely secular. There are virtually no widely-used meditation techniques that require you to compromise your beliefs to pray to any omnipresent being.

I tried meditating but I couldn't stop my thoughts - This is the most common roadblock that people erect. Meditating is not about stopping your thoughts. It is about calming down and then watching your thoughts. Trying to stop your thoughts is a sure-fire way to make yourself less relaxed, not more. Meditating is all about acceptance and letting go. Each time you find your train of thought wandering, just bring your attention back to the object of meditation (such as your breath) gently and start again.

According to Tim Ferriss, the single unifying factor in all high achievers he has interviewed for his podcast is that they all meditate regularly. Ferriss rightly points out that gradually westerners are losing the misplaced beliefs that meditation is the realm of spirituality and belief. If you strip away some of the non-core spiritual (at least in this context) aspects of meditation, what remains is a scientifically validated technique for relaxation, stress reduction and concentration enhancement.

Keep your core temperature down

OK, even I will admit this one is a bit whacky, but it is interesting enough that I wanted to include it.

Scientists have been experimenting with certain animals and have found that animals kept cooler tend to live longer. The theory is that the cooler temperatures slow down the rate of various metabolic processes and chemical reactions, theoretically slowing the aging process. For example, one study showed that by decreasing the core temperature of mice by 0.9 degrees Fahrenheit, researchers were able to extend the lifespan of mice by 20%.

The closest we have to replicating this in a practical manner in humans is through the consumption of *wasabi* – the hot horseradish used in Japanese sushi!

This is probably one for you to file away under "Useless Information", however I thought it was an interesting concept. My main problem is firstly that it doesn't seem to match up with the *Blue Zones*, which are mostly quite warm. I admit however that there could be a confounding factor – maybe the Blue Zone populations would live even longer if they pulled up sticks and moved to Greenland. My second problem is – even if this were verified, reducing your core temperature on a regular basis would be rather impractical. Short of building your own cool room or taking ice baths, it is fairly difficult to reduce you core temperature on a regular basis by any meaningful degree. One possible avenue is a drug that works similar to acetaminophen but without the glutathione-depleting aspects. As you may remember from last time you were sick and had a fever, acetaminophen can reduce body temperature a little.

If I can think of a single practical suggestion for reducing your average core body temperature it would be to switch some of your exercise focus to swimming. This could potentially kill two birds with one stone if you are also trying to manage your weight. The reduction in core temperature that accompanies swimming in cold water has been shown to dramatically increase your metabolic rate as your body works hard to bring your temperature back up to homeostasis. This is apparently the reason why Olympic swimmer Michael Phelps was able to consume such a huge number of calories each day and not gain weight. It was calculated that his energy consumption far outweighed his energy output from swimming, with the thermogenic effect of cold water the primary explanation.

Live a life of purpose

One of the great ironies of life is that many people spend their whole life working to that they can enjoy a comfortable retirement. They then reach this milestone and, lacking purpose, direction and structure to their day, they inexplicably die. For many years this has been a puzzling phenomenon. People retire and think that they will be able to just enjoy laying around all day reading the newspaper. Unfortunately for most people, our mind doesn't work that way. It needs purpose and direction to sustain it. Sometimes it almost seems as if your body takes retirement as a sign that its job here on Earth is done and it can now promptly expire.

For example a 2009 study of around 1200 elderly subjects found that those with a sense of purpose in life were half as likely to die in the five year study period as those without a sense of purpose. Half! That is an amazing figure. The study concluded *"Greater purpose in life is associated with a reduced risk of all-cause mortality among community-dwelling older persons"*

A sense of purpose is also believe to be a unifying factor in the Blue Zones which contributes to the greater life expectancy seen in these areas.

However the benefits are not just limited to the elderly. If we can just revisit stress, anxiety and depression for a moment, we will see that certain events or situation are not inherently bad – it is just that they are perceived to be negative by our own minds. If you are in a job that is incredibly demanding, depending on how you view your job, you will have a vastly different reaction on a cellular level.

Busyness does not equal stress. If you are doing what you love and you feel charged with purpose, you won't suffer the same biological consequences as someone trapped in a stressful, dead-end job.

Do what you can to give yourself a sense of purpose. Either change your situation or change how you view your situation.

Looking younger through appropriate skin care

I was initially planning to avoid mentioning skin care in this book because having "glowing" skin is not going to help you reach 100. However I have since taken some time to think about it and have changed my mind. The reason for this is that for many people, having younger looking skin makes them happy. They know that most of the invented, science-y sounding ingredients in their $100 jar of cream is not going to miraculously make them look twenty years younger. They know it is mostly marketing and placebo effect. But they don't care – because it makes them happy. The act of buying the latest cream advertised in Vanity Fair is enjoyable. The act of putting it on their skin is enjoyable. For many, this whole routine is like their own person Japanese tea ceremony.

Furthermore, I have realized that many people will be reading this book as part of a nascent personal makeover project. For these people, as well as feeling better they want to look better. And looking better makes them feel better.

Fortunately, there is one key fact that makes this a very easy section for me to write – Doing everything else in this book will be the single greatest thing they can do to achieve younger looking skin. Getting enough sleep and adopting a diet rich in omega 3 and antioxidants will do far more than most expensive skin care cream out there.

The good news also is that there are a few ingredients out there that actually work.

Firstly, we need to acknowledge that there are two types of skin aging – intrinsic and extrinsic. Intrinsic aging happens regardless of whether we look after our skin. As each year passes, there are changes to collagen and elastin fibers that eventually result in wrinkles and other signs of aging. Extrinsic aging refers to the environmental factors that accelerate the aging process of your skin. Fortunately there are things you can do to mitigate this process.

The beauty (pardon the pun) of anti-aging skin care is that all the concepts that apply to the rest of your body also apply to the skin. A large amount of the damage your skin sustains is caused by free radicals and advanced glycation end-products (AGEs). Remember the protein cross-linking I mentioned earlier that AGEs involve? That process is one of the reasons why prematurely aged skin looks more brittle and has less elasticity. So by following all the recommendations in this book regarding AGEs and antioxidants, you have already ticked a large box in terms of keeping your skin from aging prematurely.

However the number one premature ager of skin is UVA and UVB exposure from sunlight. This is where things get tricky because I believe that, as a society, we have developed the habit of avoiding sunlight due to perceived skin cancer risk, at the expense of our vitamin D status. And here is where it complicates further – one of the main processes of renewal that occurs in your skin – the production of keratinocytes – is controlled to a certain extent by vitamin D. Not complicated enough yet? Well, how about the fact that vitamin D itself has been shown to demonstrate photo-protective benefits for the skin? No problem, just put on sunscreen before you go outside so you get the vitamin D but without the skin-aging effects. Sorry – sunscreen blocks the absorption of ultraviolet light needed to trigger vitamin D production.

So, let's get this straight – You need vitamin D for a range of skin renewal and skin protection processes. You can't put on sunscreen or else you won't produce any vitamin D. So, logically you need to expose yourself to damaging ultraviolet light to get the anti-aging benefits of vitamin D. It's enough to give anyone a headache.

There are two ways to deal with this.

Firstly, carefully control both your exposure to sunlight and the areas of your body that are exposed. If you keep exposure to under twenty minutes or so, you are unlikely to suffer any real photo-damage. If you are concerned about premature aging to the skin on aesthetically important parts of your body (face, hands, neck etc.), try to get exposure to parts of your body that are not typically exposed. Here is something I experimented with in the name of this book. We have a sun lounge in our backyard. Once a day I laid down on the lounge, took my shirt off, covered my face and stayed there for around fifteen minutes or so. Theoretically, with whiter skin on the parts of your body that are not usually exposed, you should be able to produce vitamin D more effectively and require less time in the sun (*Note – this is an important point – the darker your skin, the less vitamin D you are able to produce from sunlight. This puts darker-skinned people who move to colder locations at greater risk of vitamin D deficiency*). If your skin goes red, you have stayed out too long.

Secondly, many dermatologists are now recommending a greater focus on dietary and supplemental vitamin D support instead of sun exposure. They are recommending anywhere from 4000-10,000IU per day from supplements to replace a large proportion of sun exposure. This way you will be getting all the benefits of vitamin D without the photoaging. The only downside is that your body has better control over its own vitamin D status when you are absorbing it mainly from the sun. It is able to switch off the production of vitamin D when levels are adequate. There is no risk of toxicity from sun exposure, which is one of the downsides of taking supplements. However I should also point out that there is a growing chorus of experts who have said that, unless massive doses are being taken each day, your risk of vitamin D toxicity is low. If you stick to 10,000IU and under per day, there is little risk of toxicity. However, as I have mentioned previously, ensure you add vitamin K supplements to your regime if you are taking more than a few thousand IU per day of vitamin D.

I am no expert on individual anti-aging creams. In fact, the whole beauty industry gives me an uncomfortable feeling the way it has no qualms about blatantly lying about the effectiveness of their products. However, I have dug into some research journals to separate fact from fiction. Even this is no guarantee that you will be able to avoid questionable ethics. For example, I stumbled on a paper which appeared to show a particular cream having superior anti-aging effects when compared to placebo. My excitement dimmed somewhat when I noticed down the bottom that the research study had been commissioned by the retail chain with exclusive selling rights to this particular cream!

I will risk further alienating the cosmetics industry when I tell you that by far the most effective anti-aging cream available is not even a retail product. It is only available on prescription from your doctor or dermatologist. This substance is a vitamin A retinoid known as *tretinoin* (Retin-A). What is particularly frustrating for the cosmetics industry is that they are allowed to use tretinoin in their own products, but only at concentrations so weak that they are virtually ineffective. If you want to try tretinoin you will have to get it via your doctor or dermatologist. Tretinoin has been shown to –

- Prevent and treat wrinkles effectively (don't expect miracles however)

- Prevent and treat age spots

- Assist in building collagen levels, creating a "younger-looking appearance" (this one is slightly vague for my liking)

In terms of the ingredients to look for in commercially available products, you should look for –

Ingredients that treat and prevent oxidative damage – vitamin C, green tea, idebenone, vitamin e

Ingredients that trigger skin renewal (such as collagen production) – retinol (make sure you avoid anything with *pro-retinols* like *retinyl palmitate, retinyl acetate,* and *retinyl linoleate*)

Ingredients that fill out wrinkles (temporarily lessening their appearance) - Hyaluronic Acid

Ingredients that trigger skin-cell turnover, giving a temporarily younger appearance – AHA, salicylic acid (BHA)

However probably the most overlooked way to prevent wrinkles from appearing and to temporarily lessen their appearance is to keep your skin well hydrated. Some ingredients to look for in products for both your face and body are – Sorbolene (the cheapest and the best in many cases!), products using oats or shea butter.

Conclusion

As you will probably agree, that is a potentially confusing array of methods for increasing longevity. It's a lot to take in.

Company CEOs often like to get "one-pagers" from their staff that enables them to get across the issues without having to dig deep into the background or possibly unnecessary detail. So, here is my version of a one-pager that summarizes everything you need to know in terms of increasing life expectancy –

- Avoid or reduce sources of stress

- Get enough sleep

- Don't smoke or abuse drugs (legal or otherwise). Reduce or eliminate alcohol

- Get regular exercise including cardiovascular exercise and weight training. Also ensure you include stretching and mobility-type exercise such as yoga or Pilates.

- Compulsory supplements for virtually everyone – omega 3 fatty acids (via fish oil, krill oil or even the more recent calamari oil), vitamin D, curcumin, n-acetylcysteine, alpha lipoic acid. Plus optional supplements for decreasing oxidative stress such as resveratrol – if your budget allows

- Make educated decisions regarding medication. Always consider the risk/benefit ratio. If a medication will help you live longer or reduce suffering, take it. If it causes more problems than it treats, ditch it and investigate alternatives.

- Get at least 20 minutes of sunshine on your exposed skin each day. Don't go overboard with avoiding the sun altogether due to perceived skin cancer risk. You are more likely to get cancer from avoiding the sun (and getting vitamin D deficient) than you are from 20 minutes a day of sun exposure.

- Maintain a sense of purpose. Have a reason for getting out of bed each day.

- Maintain a rich network of social connections with friends and family. Avoid spending extended periods alone. A bit of solitary introspection is healthy. Too much is considerably unhealthier.

- Keep your brain healthy with intellectually stimulating activities and optional use of nootropic supplements that modulate dopamine and acetylcholine.

- Move to a Paleo-style diet. This doesn't mean you have to go "full Paleo" and ban all dairy, grains and legumes. In my case, I still eat all of those things but in much less quantity than I used to. Don't be a fundamentalist. If wheat doesn't cause you any problems – fine – keep eating it. However remember that some problems don't occur immediately, like where some people will get an immediate stomach ache after consuming wheat. The chronic, low level inflammation that wheat causes for many will take longer to reveal itself.

- The more vegetables you eat (particularly leafy greens), the longer you will live. This is one of the undisputed aspects of diet. Everyone agrees this point, whether they are up on the latest science or whether they are those conservative old nutritionists who still recommend plenty of "whole grains". Eat more veges.

- Regarding animal protein, where possible, try to switch your focus from red meat and chicken to seafood-based options like fish, squid, oysters etc.

- Closely monitor all possible aspects of your health and get regular check-ups.

- Engage in risky behaviour with a full understanding that you are reducing your life expectancy. Each single episode of risky behaviour is like playing Russian roulette using a gun with a lot of empty chambers. As risk increases, the number of empty chambers decreases.

- Always wear a sunscreen on your face to prevent premature photoaging.

If you find all this overwhelming, you can apply Pareto's law and just focus on –

- The causes of mortality over which you have the greatest control, and;

- The most common causes of mortality

For example, if you reduce your chances of dying from either heart disease, stroke or cancer, you have dramatically increased your chances of living past 100.

I feel I also need to address what is outside of our control.

Firstly, we need to acknowledge the impact of genetic makeup. While we don't know the exact proportion of effect, reaching 100 involves genetics to a certain degree. However, with each new research study that comes out, we are increasingly seeing the focus switch to interventions which can overcome genetic shortcomings. Don't become fatalistic. Focus on what you can control to mitigate any additional risk you may have of dying from a particular cause.

Secondly we need to at least give the power of *chance* a cursory glance. Yes, you could follow everything in this guide, have the cellular age of someone twenty years younger, yet still be run over by a bus tomorrow. Without wishing to get too philosophical, yes, our lives are always hanging by a thin gossamer thread. It is actually healthy to realize this – which is why a lot of meditative focus in Buddhism is directed towards appreciating that your time is limited, so you'd better make the most of this precious human birth we have been granted. All I can say is yes, chance could take your life at any minute, but remember that risk is additive. If you add in the chances of accidental death on top of accelerated cellular aging, you have almost no chance of reaching old age whatsoever. Focus on what you can control.

Before I go, I want to stress that this book is a living document that will regularly be updated as new research emerges. If we stay on the topic of Buddhism for a moment, once the Dalai Lama was asked what he would do if science disproved any aspect of what Buddhists believe, he replied *"If scientific analysis were conclusively to demonstrate certain claims in Buddhism to be false, then we must accept the findings of science and abandon those claims."*

Likewise, if new information emerges that disproves what we now believe, I will update my position. As I have stressed many times before – don't be fundamentalist about anything. If the consensus on wheat changes, I will be the first to load up on delicious croissants. However, where I stand now, I clearly know that croissants (one of my favorite foods on the planet by the way – it's my guilty secret) and other bread products make me put on weight and I feel slightly ill after eating them.

If you think I have gotten the science wrong, made an error or something in this book has become out of date due to new research, please let me know – james@authorjameslee.com.

Above all, educate yourself and don't be afraid to experiment. In business, the key to experimentation is survival. If a company wishes to try a new strategy, this new strategy should not jeopardize the company's survival. Likewise, healthy experimentation is fine. Just be aware of the risk/benefit ratio.

January 2015 Update

What changes have occurred since I wrote this book? There have been a few worth mentioning –

1. The discovery of nicotinamide mononucleotide has certainly been one of the most notable events of recent times. Whilst things are still in the early stages, this substance is demonstrating some fascinating anti-aging properties. However unless you have a few hundred grand burning a hole in your pocket, this is still too expensive for general sale as of today. However if additional trials are positive, expect to see this substance either in pharmaceutical products or even as a supplement in the future.

2. Which leads me to my disappointment in resveratrol. Each trial that comes out lately appears to pour cold water on the early promise shown by resveratrol. It is by no means proven conclusively to be ineffective, however the early sheen has certainly rubbed off. My feeling is that resveratrol suffers from a bioavailability problem which is not unlike curcumin, so we could potentially see patented products come out which overcome this issue and enable resveratrol to slow the aging process as we first expected. At this stage, it is important to point out that there are no known safety issues, so this is no reason to throw your resveratrol in the garbage bin. However, compared to some other products, the evidence for resveratrol is, at this point in time, weaker. Pterostilbene appears to be a much better option at this stage, however until it starts to gain more widespread understanding, availability is limited.

3. Which again leads me to the rising star of anti-aging – astaxanthin. It seems like almost every day I see a new study showing a beneficial effect of this amazing substance. Many researchers now believe that astaxanthin is the single most potent anti-oxidant known. Since writing this book, I have made astaxanthin a central component of my own personal longevity prescription, along with some other stars such as curcumin. More on astaxanthin later in this book.

4. The next candidate for future anti-aging stardom is sulforaphane, the amazing substance found in broccoli. Unfortunately supplement makers still haven't

cracked the code of how to deliver pure sulforaphane in a tablet, due to the complex metabolism and conversions involved. If you see a supplement advertised as "sulforaphane", avoid it as it won't be able to give you the benefits of the natural sulforaphane found in broccoli. However the good news is that you *can* get a super-concentrated dose of sulforaphane via broccoli sprout powder, which is available from a limited number of online suppliers. Or you could do what I do and just eat lots and lots of broccoli! However remember to steam, not boil, if you want to retain the benefits of sulforaphane. Again, I will give you some more info on this later.

Part 2 - Your Brain Electric

A common experience I have when providing consulting to clients is that they often have a huge appetite for learning more about their own individual neurochemistry. You can't fix what you can't identify and in this context it means that when you understand what is happening inside your own skull a little better, it enables you to tweak and tinker using a range of substances and Behaviours.

For example, we know that a deficit in serotonin functioning can cause everything from outright major depressive disorder (MDD) to sleep disorders and even aggressive behaviour. A low dopamine state can prevent you from feeling pleasure or even just a mild lack of motivation.

However more is not always better, which is why a nuanced understanding of this topic is required. Whilst low dopamine can feel pretty crappy, if, for example, you were able to push your brain to the extreme in the other direction (i.e. – a hyper-dopaminergic state), you could create a quasi-schizophrenic state. This is why many anti-psychotic drugs used to treat schizophrenia act as dopamine antagonists, blocking the effects of this fascinating neurotransmitter. Similarly, if you were able to create a state of massive levels of serotonin, you would block the effects of dopamine (one tends to compete with the other in certain parts of the brain) and would be unable to feel pleasure (not to mention you would have a complete lack of libido – not a state desired by many!).

This is why I believe that any earnest program of biohacking and cognitive optimization must involve at least some understanding of what is occurring under the hood. As I will explain, there are identifiable differences in different neurochemical states. Understanding these differences allows you to tinker and optimize.

There is a saying in science circles which says that if someone tells you they understand quantum physics, they *don't* understand quantum physics! Similarly, if someone tells you that "serotonin is the feel-good hormone" or "dopamine is the chemical of pleasure", they *don't* understand neurochemistry. Well, maybe it is part of the story but not the whole story as both of these neurotransmitters, along with many others, are responsible for a wide range of effects throughout your brain and body.

Actually, the quantum physicals analogy is appropriate, as much of what happens inside your head operates more closely to the principles of quantum mechanics than it does to basic Newtonian physics. Rather than "if we do X then Y will occur", we have to talk the language of "action potentials", where particular chemical and electrical reactions occur without any fixed rule.

There are several reasons why I wrote this book. First and foremost, I have found that many people are interested in their own neurochemistry but are often scared off reading further by dense and boring textbooks on the topic. If you are ever having trouble sleeping, type in "serotonergic" into PubMed (where research trials and clinical reviews are published) and start reading. You will be asleep in minutes. So I want this book to serve as a tool to make what can often be a fascinating topic more accessible and entertaining.

Secondly, a sound understanding of basic neurochemistry and neurotransmission can quite often serve as an extremely useful diagnostic tool for your own particular mood or cognitive issues. Depression is an extremely common disorder, with around 5-10% of westerners clinically depressed at any one time and an amazing one out of four American women over the age of 50 currently on antidepressants.

When the average person visits their doctor suffering depression, they will invariably leave with a script for a drug which increases serotonin in the brain. This is despite the fact that there are a range of different neurochemical issues which can cause depression (or at least are associated with depression) and only some of which involve serotonin directly. The good news is that depression caused by low serotonin and depression caused by low dopamine or noradrenaline is usually strikingly different and fairly easy to identify if you know what you are looking for. So in this book I will give you all the information you need to know so you can easily tell the difference.

However I should also make another important point – *You are more than your neurotransmitters*. There is often a tendency to oversimplify what happens inside your head and to explain everything in terms of serotonin or dopamine. This is largely a construct of pharmaceutical companies whose self-serving "chemical imbalance" theory of anxiety and depression has become the default explanation when something goes awry inside our heads. There is no single illness called "depression" or "anxiety" and there are countless variations of each (as I will explain later). For example, whilst many people have depression caused by a lack of serotonin (or impaired serotonergic functioning), many do not. Depression can be caused by faulty thinking, life stressors, low dopamine, low noradrenaline, too much glutamate, thyroid problems and sleep disorders, to name but a few.

Considering this complexity, it is no surprise that there is no single treatment for all kinds of depression and anxiety. You have probably hear of SSRI drugs (*selective serotonin reuptake inhibitors* such as *Prozac*) which work by inhibiting the process by which your brain removes serotonin from the synapse (Don't worry, I will explain what synapses are also) and therefore keeping levels higher than they would have been. Sounds simple right? Well, did you know that there is another antidepressant drug called *Stablon* (tianeptine) which is a selective serotonin reuptake *enhancer*? Yes, that's right. Stablon does the exact opposite thing in your brain yet it also treats depression for some people.

First up I will give you a quick and dirty introduction to neurotransmission (Don't worry, I promise I won't bore you!) and then I will go into more detail on some of the main neurotransmitters in the brain which are relevant for mood disorders such as anxiety and depression.

Oh, and one more thing. As I have written a range of books and guides on various topics directly related to brain health and brain optimization, whenever I mention a topic covered in greater detail in one of my other books, I will hyperlink it so you can click on the link and check it out to see if it interests you. Remember each book you purchase helps me make the repayments on my Maserati (Well, it's an 8 year old Mitsubishi, but I guess if you squint really hard it might look kinda Italian).

OK. Let's begin.

What is "neurotransmission"?

Neurotransmission is the mechanism your brain uses to send messages and trigger reactions by a kind of electrical transmission. Imagine a long line of people that stretches for miles. If someone at one end of the line wanted to get a message to the person at the other end, they would have one choice – *Chinese whispers*! That is how your brain communicates except that instead of people, you have individual neurons (brain cells) and instead of a whisper, each neuron releases a certain type of neurotransmitter to get the message across to the other neuron.

There is a gap between each neuron which is known as a *synapse* (or the *synaptic cleft*) and neurotransmitters are your brain's way of getting the message across the gap. The neurotransmitters are stored in vesicles (think of vesicles like little pouches) on the pre-synaptic neuron (the neuron sending the message is known as the *pre-synaptic neuron* and the neuron receiving the message is, unsurprisingly, known as the *post-synaptic neuron*).

Think of your neurotransmitters as keys which then need to open the right locks on the post-synaptic neuron. These locks are known as receptors. When a neurotransmitter binds to the receptor it triggers a reaction which then can often cascade through your nervous system using a kind of Chinese whispers system I mentioned earlier.

If you imagine a chain of neurons for a moment, it is easy to provide a simplified visualization. Imagine the first neuron in the chain. It sends out a message using, say, serotonin, by sending it out via an axon (imagine a squid with tentacles – the axon is a tentacle that sends messages to nearby neurons). The serotonin will then bind to a specific receptor (called the *5-ht receptor*) on a tentacle on the receiving neuron called a dendrite. Axons send the message and dendrites receive.

There are a multitude of neurotransmitters and they are generally classified as either excitatory or inhibitory. This doesn't necessarily mean that they make you "excited" (although neurotransmitters such as norepinephrine and dopamine certainly can), but means that they increase the chance that the neuron will then go on to fire an *action potential*. I would be at risk of boring you if I spent too much time getting into the detail of action potential, however suffice to say that when a neurotransmitter binds to a receptor, it is no guarantee of a predictable reaction, but a "potential" reaction. The key is for the neurochemical messenger received by the neuron to surpass a particular threshold of electrical activity. If it does so, an action potential will be triggered and if not, it won't.

The main excitatory neurotransmitters are glutamate, acetylcholine and norepinephrine (and epinephrine), while the primary inhibitory neurotransmitters are GABA and serotonin. Serotonin is actually a complicated one and is more accurately called a neuromodulator because, depending on the context, can be either excitatory or inhibitory. Despite this, by far the most common neurotransmitters in your nervous system are glutamate and GABA.

Modulating Neurotransmitter Activity with Drugs and Natural Substances

If you are reading this book, I am fairly confident that you have more than just a passing interest in fixing your own neurotransmitter activity or at least, optimizing it. This can be a complicated topic so I have taken great pains to simplify this topic in the clearest possible terms. I also endeavor to be refreshingly clear of bias or a "fundamentalist" position. This is not a book where you will be told about the "evils" of "big pharma" or the apparently "magical" properties of various herbs and concoctions. Similarly, I will not try to tell you that all natural medicine is useless and that drugs are the only answer. You don't have to pick one or the other. You have the option of getting the best of both worlds.

However, I will be clear on one fairly reliable law of neurochemistry – If you are suffering from a severe issue (such as severe depression or anxiety), you will almost certainly require some kind of pharmacological assistance (along with everything else you will need to do to heal). For severe mental illness, supplements and herbal medicines don't cut it and those people recommending you stop your medication and go on a natural medicine are being reckless with other peoples' health. Likewise, for mild issues (mild anxiety, feeling sub-par and the like), antidepressants don't perform any better than a placebo. If you are in this scenario, it is likely that troubling side-effects would outweigh any benefits and you would be more likely to see results with particular natural therapies, along with the single greatest healer of neurochemical problems – exercise! (More on this later...)

Now, if, for some reason, you would like to increase levels of neurotransmitters such as serotonin, dopamine or noradrenaline, there are a limited number of pathways you can use to achieve this. This also leads to one of my bugbears with some proponents of natural therapies, who can sometimes make it seem like herbal medicines treat depression via some unique and separate pathway than that used by drugs. Popular herbal antidepressants such as St. John's Wort and Rhodiola Rosea treat depression the same way that certain drugs do, so the "natural" tag is, in some ways, a misnomer.

So, what are these ways we can increase levels of neurotransmitters? Let's use serotonin as an example to explain the various ways we can boost levels –

1. **Inhibit the "re-uptake" process**
   When serotonin has done its job and triggered an action potential, your brain has a system for recycling it. There is a molecule known as the SERT (serotonin transporter) which acts like a bus that picks up the serotonin and takes it back to its "home base" neuron for processing. By blocking the action of SERT, more serotonin can build up in the synapse and hopefully, lead to improved mood or reduced anxiety.

This is how the popular SSRIs (selective serotonin re-uptake inhibitors such as Prozac and Zoloft) work. The main advantage of SSRIs over older antidepressants is that SSRIs are more "selective" (which should come as no surprise considering the name...) and therefore cause less side-effects. Some of the older antidepressants are subject to side-effects which can range from mildly troubling to life-threatening. However SSRIs are not without their own troubling side-effects, which include a constellation of problems from sexual dysfunction to diarrhea.

The older class of antidepressants known as tricyclics also work in this way. This class, which includes drugs such as amitriptyline and clomipramine, is notorious for being un-selective (hence SSRIs are known as selective because they essentially target serotonin only) and therefore comes with a range of side-effects such as drowsiness. However their non-selectivity means that they are useful for a range of other applications such as amitriptyline's use for treating neuropathic pain and insomnia.

2. Block the action of the enzyme that breaks down serotonin

Another way serotonin is recycled after it has done its job is via an enzyme known as monoamine oxidase (MAO), which breaks down serotonin (as well as dopamine and noradrenaline) via an enzymatic process. Similarly to SSRIs, if you block this process, the serotonin doesn't get broken down at the same rate and then has a chance to build up in the synapse.

Drugs that do this are called MAOIs (monoamine oxidase inhibitors) and were an older class of medications that are rarely used these days due to safety concerns. The main problem with MAOIs is that they require dietary restrictions. If someone taking a MAOI consumes food or drink high in tyramine (such as aged cheese), it can trigger a massive spike in blood pressure and can lead to death. So it's not surprising that these have been largely ditched since the advent of SSRIs, which are virtually impossible to overdose on or accidentally kill yourself with.

That said, many experts believe that MAOIs remain the most effective antidepressant drugs to this day and they are therefore used occasionally with those who don't respond to other drugs. If you are in a deep dark hole the, according to certain experts, your best bet is either MAOIs or ECT (electroconvulsive therapy).

3. Stimulating the receptor

Substances known as receptor agonists can artificially activate receptors, triggering the effects that would occur if the neurotransmitter itself did the job. For certain receptor types, this is a simple proposition, whereas for others, things get a little complicated. For example, opiate drugs such as morphine and codeine function as opiate agonists, mimicking the action of natural endorphins and consequently reducing pain. The class of anti-anxiety (and sleep) medications known as benzodiazepines (such as Xanax, Temazepam and Valium) act as GABA receptor agonists and therefore calm you down.

However serotonin receptors are a little more complicated and this is the reason why there are no effective antidepressants which operate primarily as serotonin receptor agonists. This is because there are a range of sub-types of the serotonin receptor and each sub-type has different effects when activated. For example, activating the 5-HT$_{1A}$ receptor can reduce anxiety (such as the drugs buspirone and trazodone), whereas activating 5-HT$_{2A}$ (such as psychedelics such as LSD do) can make you believe that there is a clown in your closet who wants you dead. Or alternatively, activating 5-HT$_{1B}$ (as the triptan class of drugs do) will treat migraines and cluster headaches. If you go messing around with serotonin, you'd better make sure you target the right receptor!

Then there are inverse agonists which agonies the receptor to trigger the exact opposite effect as a direct agonist would.

In case you were wondering, yes, serotonin and other neurotransmitters are classified as agonists of their relevant receptors.

4. **Blocking the receptor**

A receptor antagonist (or a receptor blocker) occupies the receptor and prevents the endogenous (natural/non-pharmacological) neurotransmitter from doing its job.

Of all the various ways you can modulate receptor activity, antagonism can be the most confusing to understand because of the different ways that different types of receptors (and neurotransmitters) respond to antagonism. For example, the common class of anti-hypertensive drugs (to reduce blood pressure) known as beta-blockers block the beta-adrenal receptors and reduce blood pressure (by reducing adrenal activation of those receptors. However, there are a class of antidepressants which act as serotonin receptor antagonists (such as mirtazapine). How can a drug which blocks serotonin treat depression? This is actually a very long story and I would run the real risk of boring you to death so I will give you the "digest" version. Firstly, there are many researchers who dispute whether serotonin receptor antagonists even increase serotonergic neurotransmission. This is backed up by the fact that antagonists such as mirtazapine don't cause any of the effects typically associated with increased serotonin (such as serotonin syndrome or sexual dysfunction). However other researchers believe that antagonists increase serotonin by blocking the sub-types which increase anxiety and depression and thereby increasing activity of the unaffected sub-types.

5. **Stimulating the release of the neurotransmitter (or inhibiting storage – however you wish to call it)**

The other way we can increase levels of serotonin and other neurotransmitters is to force the presynaptic neuron to release its stores. Imagine the serotonin is sitting in a bag hanging from the roof. This is the equivalent of squeezing on the bag to force the contents out.

In the case of serotonin, the most potent releasing agent is the drug ecstasy which basically drains your brain of not only serotonin but also tryptophan, the amino acid precursor. This is why, unsurprisingly, you feel rather depressed after an ecstasy "trip". As a side note, next time someone tries to tell you that depression has nothing to do with serotonin, you can helpfully point out ecstasy, where serotonin depletion causes a perfect analogue of depression (albeit for a few days only). (Note – As I will mention repeatedly, this does not mean that all depression is caused by serotonin. There is depression cause by low dopamine and a multitude of other causes. However depression related to low serotonin is undeniably common. I should also point out that we don't yet know whether low serotonin causes depression or is the result of depression. That's how complicated this picture is!)

The most common releasing agents are the amphetamine class of drugs and the ADHD medication methylphenidate (Ritalin). Amphetamines powerfully trigger the release of noradrenaline, dopamine and serotonin. Considering such powerful action on all three of your key mood related neurotransmitters (with the exception of opiate receptors perhaps), it is not hard to see why drugs like methamphetamine (meth) are so addictive.

In general, releasing agents are fraught with danger because they tend to rob future neurotransmitters to feed the present. For example, reuptake inhibitors gradually increase serotonin over time, whereas releasing agents dump everything into the synapse, leaving none for tomorrow. This means, as a general rule regarding depression and anxiety, releasing agents make you feel much better today and then much worse tomorrow as your brain just can't replenish levels of neurotransmitters quickly enough to keep up.

What about "natural" substances?

If you are considering a natural alternative to a particular drug, you need to bear in mind that, in general, most supplements and herbs will work in the same basic ways mentioned above. And when you read about a particular supplement being "milder" with less side-effects, sometimes it can mean that there are no positive effects either.

Essentially, natural antidepressants work as either mild SSRIs or mild MAOIs, with often conflicting research as to which. For example, researchers are currently divided as to whether St. John's Wort is an SSRI or a MAOI. At the end of the day, this is relatively unimportant. More pertinent is whether sometime works or not. The only exception to this is when you are suffering from low dopamine. SSRIs tend to suppress dopaminergic function whereas MAOIs give all three mood-related monoamine neurotransmitters a boost. So if low dopamine is an issue, you would either need to focus on a supplement that purely works on dopamine (such as mucuna pruriens) or a MAOI like rhodiola rosea.

Serotonin

What is it and what does it do?

Serotonin is a monoamine neurotransmitter involved in a range of functions including mood, appetite, sleep, digestion. Serotonin is known as the "feel-good hormone", however the majority of all serotonin in your body is located in your gut, where it drives the process of digestion.

What are the symptoms of low serotonin?

Low levels of serotonin are strongly associated with the following symptoms –

- Low mood
- Anxiety
- Sleeping problems (insomnia, poor quality sleep)
- Aggression
- Increased pain
- Digestive problems (constipation, diarrhoea, stomach pains)

How do I fix my problems with serotonin?

The good news is that issues related to low serotonin are relatively easy to fix with either drugs, supplements or cognitive and behavioral changes. However it is not all good news and there are a few things you should note.

Serotonin problems are slow to fix and just replenishing serotonin doesn't cure depression.

One of the great mysteries of pharmacology is why it takes up to 3 months to improve when someone takes an antidepressant like an SSRI, as serum levels of serotonin (measured via metabolites) only take around 3 days to normalise. This is due to several reasons.

When you restore serotonin levels via drug therapy, it triggers (perhaps indirectly) a gradual healing process that can take a long time. Firstly, we have the issue of receptor down-regulation and up-regulation. When there is low serotonergic activity for a long period of time, serotonin receptors up-regulate, which means, they become much better at utilising the limited supply of serotonin more efficiently. However, when you start taking an SSRI, it triggers an interesting process which many researchers believe is the reason why a small minority of people commit suicide shortly after starting an antidepressant.

The first thing that happens is that your brain, through special receptors, senses that there is ample serotonin available and throttles back production and release. This can then send someone into a temporary yet intensely unpleasant black hole as their brain then starts to adjust. Beginning an antidepressant is often a case of "two steps forward, one step back". It is fascinating that most people I have dealt with or followed on various discussion forums have followed an almost identical timeline –

Day 1-3 – Increased anxiety as the drug gives an almost stimulant effect.

Day 3-7 – Happier than they have been since becoming ill. Sometimes almost euphoric as their serotonin levels spike.

Week 2-3 – Mood drops again as the brain throttles serotonergic activity. This can either be a minor drop in mood or suicidally bad, depending on the person. If this is you, the key point to raise here is not to give up hope. I think many people just assume they are about to fall back into a black hole again and never come out. This kind of thinking could reasonably lead to suicidal thoughts.

Week 3-12 – Gradual improvement and by the third month will start to think of themselves as "back to normal".

However as you probably know, not everyone responds to antidepressants and this leads to the second complicating point with treating problems with serotonin. Firstly, as I have already mentioned, not all depression is caused by serotonergic issues. So someone with a kind of *anhedonic* (inability to feel pleasure) depression caused by low dopamine would not show the same recovery timeline as the example above. This is one of the problems with the modern obsession drug companies have with serotonin. For example, the only option at present for someone with depression caused by low dopamine is either an old-school MAOI or the smoking cessation aid bupropion (*Wellbutrin* when used for depression and *Zyban* when used for quitting smoking).

Secondly, even if serotonin is behind your depression (or anxiety), it is not simply a case of filling up the tank and away we go. There are countless ways your serotonin system can get out of whack. Some of the more common are –

1. Not enough serotonin being released by the presynaptic neuron
2. Your re-uptake process is too quick, leaving too little serotonin in the synapse
3. Your MAO activity is too high, breaking down serotonin too quickly
4. You are not consuming enough tryptophan in your diet, so your brain cannot produce enough serotonin
5. You are consuming enough tryptophan however your body is inefficient at converting it into serotonin
6. You are consuming a diet high in tyrosine relative to tryptophan. Tyrosine is the amino acid precursor to dopamine and noradrenaline and it competes with tryptophan to cross the blood brain barrier (the barrier which protects your brain from various alien substances).

And this is just looking at the biochemical pathways. Possibly more relevant is looking at the various cognitive and behavioral processes that send serotonin levels lower. A stressful life or a dead-end job will mess up serotonin more swiftly than any of the pathways mentioned above. More on this in a moment.

So naturally, depending on your particular quirks, different treatments will have different outcomes. For example, on many forums you will see people claiming that tryptophan or 5-htp (5-htp is another supplement which is one step closer to serotonin, biochemically) are effective antidepressants. If low levels of tryptophan are behind your particular issues, then this will be the case. However if you are depressed, yet have no issues with tryptophan, taking these types of supplements will be unlikely to help.

So this process can become one of trial and error as you experiment with what works and what doesn't work. As I mention many times, I am always about simplification and distilling everything down to key points, so I would like to summarise the process of fixing serotonergic issues like this –

1. Fix the neurochemistry via drugs or supplements. If you are suffering from mild depression or anxiety, look towards supplements. If you are suffering from moderate to severe depression or anxiety, consider pharmacological options.

2. Fix the behaviours that suppress or deplete serotonin
3. Fix the faulty thinking that suppresses or depletes serotonin.

Drug-based options

By far the most common way people boost serotonin is via SSRI antidepressants, however there are a few different ways we can increase levels of serotonin.

Selective Serotonin Re-Uptake Inhibitors (SSRIs)

SSRIs are popular for good reason. They are safe and relatively effective. They are therefore typically your doctor's first option when they suspect you have low serotonin. However I should point out that they are far from perfect. As mentioned earlier, they only work for some people and for others the side-effects can be unbearable (yet others experience either mild side-effects or none whatsoever).

The most common side effects of SSRIs are –

- Sexual dysfunction (lack of libido, problems achieving an erection and inability to orgasm)
- Sleep disturbances (These tend to be more common at the start of therapy)
- Blunted mood – This means that you feel a bit flat or don't get excited about anything. As SSRIs tend to keep people in a narrower mood band (thus preventing severe mood swing), this is not surprising.

It should also be pointed out that, for some people, coming off SSRIs (and other antidepressants also) can be hellish. If and when you need to stop SSRI therapy, you need to taper off the drug very, very slowly to minimise discontinuation syndrome.

Another thing to bear in mind is that, whilst all SSRIs work in roughly the same way, different people respond to different types, so sometimes some trial and error is required. You only have to type in (for example) "Lexapro user reviews" into Google to see this in action. For some, Lexapro changes their life and cures their depression, whereas for others it either does nothing or puts them through hell. Same goes for all of the SSRIs, so you can see how important it can often be to try a different one if the one you start with doesn't work. Just because you read someone on a forum claim that one particular SSRI is the "best", that doesn't mean the same will apply in your case.

The main SSRIs used today are –

- **Lexapro** (escitalopram)
- **Cipralex** (citalopram) (*Note – Escitalopram is the updated version of citalopram, however it doesn't necessarily mean that in your case escitalopram will work better. However in general, these two are virtually identical in terms of effects, with escitalopram having a slightly better side-effect profile*)
- **Zoloft** (sertraline)
- **Paxil** (paroxetine)
- **Prozac** (fluoxetine)

There is also another, related class known as SNRIs (serotonin and noradrenaline re-uptake inhibitors) which act in the same manner as SSRIs but also have effects on noradrenaline. The two main available SNRIs are –

- **Venlafaxine** (Effexor)

- **Desvenlafaxine** (Pristiq – A long half-life version of Effexor which enables you to only have to take one per day and it lasts until the next day)
- **Cymbalta** (duloxetine)

Again, whether you need an SSRI or an SNRI will largely come down to trial and error, however some doctors have found that, due to the extra effects on noradrenaline, SNRIs can be helpful where there is a lack of energy. On the other hand, in cases where there is already anxiety present, SNRIs can sometimes make the situation worse.

Tricyclics

The best way to think of these older class of antidepressants is like a "less specific SNRI". Whereas SNRIs can, fairly cleanly, target serotonin and noradrenaline only, tricyclics affect many other systems in the brain at the same time. This can be good and bad.

The main benefit of tricyclics' messy effects is that they can then be used to treat other conditions which respond to one of these effects. For example, amitriptyline blocks neuropathic pain signals so can be used to treat conditions such as fibromyalgia. Amitriptyline (along with several other tricyclics) also acts as a sedating antihistamine so can be used as a sleep aid.

Unfortunately it is not all good news. The greatest single difference between tricyclics and SSRIs is that, if you were insane enough to consume an entire packet (or jar) of SSRIs, you would probably live. If you did the same with tricyclics, you would probably die. In large doses, tricyclics are cardiotoxic, which, as you probably guessed, means they are not good for your heart in higher doses. They also come with a jaw-dropping long list of side-effects such as sedation and weight gain. These side-effects are not to be sniffed at and cause many people to stop taking them.

The other obvious problem is, because they increase serotonin and noradrenaline at the same time, if you want to just raise serotonin, most of them lack sufficient specificity to do this. That said, some of them (such as clomipramine) are significantly potent at increasing serotonin but less so for noradrenaline, so there are options within the class.

Tricyclics are serious drugs. They are not drugs to take if you are feeling "a little off" or looking for a "pick me up". They are potent drugs with a range of side-effects. However on the flipside, for some they can be lifesavers. Particularly those that haven't responded to SSRIs for whatever reason. For example, many experts believe that, despite the advent of SSRIs, tricyclics like clomipramine, imipramine and amitriptyline remain the most effective antidepressants available. You just have to pay the piper in terms of side-effects.

Serotonin releasing agents

As mentioned earlier, serotonin releasing agents are, in general, not sustainable options for increasing levels of serotonin as they tend to dump serotonin into your synapses at the expense of tomorrow. This is why they are not typically used as antidepressants. Oh, and there is the small issue of the most potent serotonin releaser – MDMA (ecstasy) being illegal. There is considerable debate as to whether MDMA has a role to play in legal pharmacotherapy however. Proponents (including some psychotherapists) believe that MDMA can be helpful in certain therapeutic circumstances. Other researchers point out that, in (extremely) high doses, MDMA has been shown to be neurotoxic for mice – and there are more than a few ex-ravers out there who have fried their serotonin receptors after years of abusing this drug. The truth probably lies somewhere in the middle. In fact, in the UK a few years back, Professor David Nutt (who was the government's chief advisor on drugs and drug policy) was sacked for suggesting that MDMA was less harmful than alcohol!

The only legal serotonin releasing agent available (the pain reliever tramadol) is also fraught with danger as it also has a mild opiate agonist action, making it potentially addictive for some. I actually have a vaguely controversial opinion regarding tramadol. It is one of the few legally available drugs which you can take and it improves your mood within a few hours. As you know, antidepressants take weeks to lift your mood. This is because tramadol does a few things as the same time, making it quite an interesting drug. Among other things it acts as a –

- Serotonin releasing agent (improving mood)
- Noradrenaline re-uptake inhibitor (gives you energy and lifts mood)
- Opiate agonist (dulls both mental and physical pain)
- NMDA antagonist (NMDA antagonists are the latest subject of research into new antidepressants as certain NMDA antagonists such as ketamine have been shown to lift depression in hours, not weeks!)

I believe there is a role to play for a drug like tramadol, if respected appropriately and only in very specific circumstances. There is a growing band of people claiming that when nothing else worked, tramadol lifted them out of their dark hole. However I should also point out that there is an equally large group of people telling of the horrors of quitting either large doses or long term use. This is another drug not to be trifled with and I am still not convinced of its effectiveness as a long term treatment for depression, due to the serotonin releasing properties.

Serotonin receptor antagonists and agonists

The theory behind these drugs is quite seductive and would appear to suggest that this is a promising way to increase levels of serotonin. However, unfortunately, I, along with many researchers and clinicians remain unconvinced as to the ability of antagonists and agonists to increase levels of serotonin.

There are several pieces of key evidence that show us why this is the case. Firstly, this class of drug is relatively ineffective for treating severe depression, anxiety or obsessive compulsive disorder (OCD). This is particularly the case with OCD as there is a clear relationship between the potency of a particular drug at increasing levels of serotonin and its ability to treat OCD. For example, probably the best drug for OCD is clomipramine, which is also one of the most potent agents available for increasing serotonin. While antagonists and agonists can be useful additions to an SSRI for depression or anxiety (For example – mirtazapine is fantastic for improving sleep and reducing sexual dysfunction for those on an SSRI), they are rarely a doctor's first or central option for treating these conditions.

Secondly, this class of drug does not display any of the tell-tale signs typically associated with serotonergic drugs. This is a point often repeated by respected researcher Dr Ken Gillman, who points out that it is impossible to give yourself serotonin syndrome by taking large doses of mirtazapine, or combining mirtazapine with other serotonergic drugs. As Dr Gillman points out, increasing serotonin is associated with reliable symptoms such as sexual dysfunction, however mirtazapine has the exact *opposite* effect and can actually be a *treatment* for sexual dysfunction!

So in general, if you are looking at increasing levels of serotonin, there are much better options. In the example of mirtazapine, the only exception I can think of is where low serotonin is being caused by sleep dysfunction or not eating properly. As mirtazapine is a wonderful sleep aid (mainly by increasing slow wave/deep sleep) and can make you eat like a horse, it could indirectly contribute to normalising serotonin this way.

Natural and drug-free options for boosting serotonin

When used correctly and in the right context, natural serotonin boosters can be a fantastic option for gently increasing levels over time. My book Chill Pills and Mood Food was entirely dedicated to this topic. However the problem is that often they are not used for the right reasons or in the right occasions.

Let me restate my views on this topic – If you are severely depressed, forget about using supplements and herbs. They won't help enough. Severe depression (particularly with any suicidal ideation) is not something to mess around with. Almost always, severe depression will respond best to a combination of medication, CBT (cognitive behavioral therapy) and physical exercise. Then, if your doctor agrees, once you are able to come off the medication, you could consider a mild, natural option as a kind of "maintenance therapy" to keep serotonin levels up. On the flipside, medication is complete overkill for mild depression and anxiety. This is where natural options shine. If you are feeling a bit flat or out of sorts, natural options (along with physical exercise of course!) can be wonderful for getting you back in the game. Medications come with a range of side-effects that could make you even more depressed, whereas if you are severely depressed, these side-effects are a small price to pay for recovery.

This is such a basic state of affairs that I am always shocked to read fundamentalist views by both sides of this debate. On one side you have homeopaths telling severely depressed "patients" to stop taking their medication – often with disastrous effects. On the other side you have doctors who think that anything "natural" is all just hocus pocus. The truth lies, as it usually does in most cases, somewhere in the middle of this debate.

In terms of natural options, there are a few gold-standard supplements which are already widely used, along with one or two newer options which are beginning to gain recognition.

St. John's Wort (Hypericum)

St. John's Wort is the undisputed king of herbal antidepressants for good reason. It potently increases levels of serotonin, has a long history of widespread use (making clinical studies more statistically significant) and is associated with none of the severe side-effects usually associated with pharmacological antidepressants.

St. John's Wort (or *hypericum perforatum*) is a perennial flowering herb native to Europe and some parts of Asia and Africa. It is easily recognised due to its beautiful yellow flowers. Yes, the yellow flowers have nothing to do with how it works as an antidepressant however if you are an avid gardener in the right geography, I highly recommend trying to grow St. John's Wort - it looks amazing in my own garden!

St. John's Wort has an impressive body of individual research studies and meta-analyses (where groups of studies are pooled together for better statistical significance) backing its use for mild to moderate depression, including -

- A 1995 meta-analysis of twelve individual trials founds that hypericum was significantly superior to a placebo (an "inert" sugar pill with no active ingredients) and as effective as modern pharmaceuticals at relieving depression. (This study didn't say whether it was severe or mild depression)

- A 1996 meta-analysis found that hypericum was almost three times more effective than placebo, with an efficacy that matched tricyclic antidepressants for the treatment of mild to moderate depression. Not only this, but hypericum was found to be significantly safer and with much milder side-effects.

- A more recent meta-analysis with stricter criteria was a little more subdued, albeit still with a positive outcome. This trial found that hypericum was 1.5 times as effective as placebo, but also concluded that hypericum was as effective as tricyclic drugs.

- Another study concluded that, while hypericum was effective for treating mild to moderate depression, it was slightly less effective than tricyclic drugs.

- A 1999 study found that hypericum was as effective as Prozac (fluoxetine) for the treatment of mild to moderate depression in the elderly.

The other major component of hypericum's mode of action is its ability to also concurrently treat the biomarkers of chronic stress. Stress and depression go hand in hand. It is often after a period of unrelenting stress that depression can result. Hypericum has been testing on rodents, where they are given hypericum before being subjected to various stressful situations (as an aside, everyone should take a moment to thank all these poor rodents that suffer so that we might not). In all the various measurements of stress response, hypericum has been shown to reduce the biomarkers of stress, such as cortisol levels.

Depression and chronic stress is also often associated with disturbances in the HPA (hypothalamus pituitary adrenal) axis, your brain's (and body's) system for dealing with stress. Hypericum has also been shown to positively modulate that HPA axis, leading to amelioration of certain aspects of acute and chronic stress.

It is important to note that a large number of people who start drug therapy soon quit due to intolerable side-effects. In many cases, these side-effects eventually settle down and fade, however for many people it is too hard to bear and they quit. Natural therapies such as hypericum have a much gentler start-up period, which means that, although it can take a little longer to have noticeable effects, people are unlikely to quit due to side-effects. I should also point out that this longer start-up period is another reason why natural options are not appropriate for more severe cases. If someone is severely depressed or even suicidal, their physician needs to choose the therapy that will pull them out of their deep, dark hole the most quickly. Unfortunately, I would never, ever recommend natural therapies in such acute cases. If this describes you, please put down this eBook and seek immediate, professional attention. There are powerful, effective treatments that can quickly treat your current condition.

Unfortunately there is no consensus as to exactly how hypericum exerts its beneficial effects on depression. Some researchers have claimed that it works as an SSRI, while others have indicated that it works as a MAOI. An *in-vitro* (i.e. - in a laboratory test-tube, not in an animal or human) study in 1994 found that hypericum clearly inhibited the action of monoamine oxidase when used at high doses. Similarly, studies conducted in 1997 and 1998 using even higher doses found that hypericum works at least partially as a MAOI. The problem with these high-dose studies is that they found no inhibition of monoamine oxidase using clinically relevant doses (i.e. - doses which roughly approximate what a person would typically take). So, while we know that hypericum functions as MAOI to at least some extent, it is unclear from these studies whether it functions as a MAOI at the dosages people are likely to take.

Likewise, several German studies in the 1990s found that hypericum inhibits the re-uptake of serotonin, norepinephrine and dopamine in-vitro, in a similar fashion to pharmaceutical antidepressants.

Animal studies have also all found a variety of effects, with no clear indication of a single mechanism underlying how exactly hypericum works. However the key point to draw from these and other studies is that hypericum consistently increases levels of serotonin, norepinephrine and dopamine in the brain. It's just that the relative degree to which each of these monoamines is increased or the proposed mechanism differs between studies. Of these, it appears as if serotonin is most affected, which is why I have included hypericum in this section.

While hypericum is generally an effective and potent natural antidepressant, it has one major downside - it affects how your body metabolises a variety of drugs. In fact, hypericum appears to affect almost any drug that is metabolised in the liver. Of particular concern is the impact on the blood-thinning drug warfarin. Depending on the drug, hypericum can either increase or decrease the effectiveness of the particular medication. Therefore, if you are on any drugs at all, you need to clear things with your doctor before taking hypericum. In general however, I usually recommend that, if someone is taking any other medication, to first investigate curcumin and/or rhodiola rosea, as these don't have the same effects on other drugs

The only other potential side effect of note is increased photosensitivity. In a practical sense, this means that some people can become sunburned much more quickly than otherwise would have been the case if they were not taking hypericum. So I think it would be warranted to take a little extra precaution regarding sun exposure if you are taking hypericum.

Also, I should point out that you should never combine hypericum with pharmaceutical antidepressants or any other drug that increases levels of serotonin, norepinephrine or dopamine. This can, in rare cases, lead to a life-threatening condition called serotonin syndrome. If in doubt, discuss with your primary care physician.

Rhodiola Rosea

Rhodiola is a supplement I have been passionate about for a long time now, due to its unique mechanism of action and wide-ranging effects. Along with curcumin, rhodiola is one of my picks for supplements which will become increasingly well-known over the next ten years or so.

As with hypericum and curcumin, I have chosen to include rhodiola in the section on serotonin as that is where there appears to be the most potent effects. However each of these also increases dopamine, so in mild cases where both dopamine and serotonin are lowered, these three supplements can all be great options.

Rhodiola rosea is an herbal supplement which has been used for decades in Russian-block countries to treat what they refer to as 'nervous disorders', which encapsulates a range of conditions including stress, anxiety and depression. However it has only recently risen to prominence in the West. Rhodiola rosea (also known as golden root or arctic root, among other things) is a plant that grows in cold areas of the northern hemisphere and is most commonly associated with countries such as Russia and the other countries of the former USSR and has been reputedly used extensively by the Russian military to promote endurance.

In terms of prominence in the west, rhodiola rosea still lags far behind St. John's Wort, which enjoys far more popularity and widespread use. This is a pity, because rhodiola has a few advantages over St. John's Wort (which I will get to in a moment).

Rhodiola rosea belongs to a class of herbs known as adaptogens. Adaptogens are substances which restore homeostasis in the body. So if, for example, you are too wired and anxious, an adaptogen will calm you down. If you are lethargic and lacking energy, an adaptogen will give you energy.

Quite often, I am rather suspicious of adaptogens and the theory that underpins this class of supplements. There are quite a few natural therapies marketed as adaptogens which have very poor research-based evidence backing their use. However rhodiola is one herbal medicine where there is not only a large body of anecdotal reports verifying the adaptogenic effects, but a good theoretical potential mechanism that would explain the effects.

By increasing levels of serotonin, norepinephrine and dopamine, rhodiola functions in a very similar way to a pharmaceutical antidepressant. If you are *anxious depressed* (high stress, high anxiety, poor sleep) and you take an antidepressant (such as an SSRI, tricyclic or MAOI) you will usually slowly begin to calm down and relax over time. If you are suffering from a more lethargic depression (low energy, hypersomnia, lack of motivation) and you take the same antidepressant, you will gradually start to spark up and feel more energetic. It is for this reason that, when people talk of the adaptogenic properties of rhodiola, what I believe they are really referring to is its ability to act as an antidepressant by increasing levels of the three primary monoamines.

Due to the fact that rhodiola increases levels of all three monoamines (as it acts as a MAOI), it tends to be a little more "activating" than St. John's Wort. Not surprisingly, I have therefore found it more helpful in cases of lethargic depression, rather than anxious depression.

The beauty of several antidepressant supplements such as rhodiola and curcumin, is that they function as MAOIs but without the dangerous dietary risks. This is important to note, because without the danger component, MAOIs are excellent for treating depression due to their broad range of action.

Due to the comparative lack of drug interactions, I usually recommend rhodiola rosea as the first option for treating depression if someone decides to go down the natural route. As it is a slightly newer supplement in the west, there isn't as much research yet compared to St. John's Wort, however what research is available has been generally positive. In particular, multiple rodent trials have demonstrated a clear ability to reduce some of the mental and physical effects of stress.

Apart from the fact that rhodiola works on all three monoamines compared to St. John's Wort which just affects serotonin, rhodiola has another advantage – it doesn't interact with other medications in the same way that St. John's Wort does. So if you are taking other medication and your doctor confirms that St. John's Wort could be a problem, give rhodiola some consideration.

Magnesium

Up until a few years ago, I had always thought that magnesium helped treat anxiety for one reason - *muscles need magnesium to relax*. They use calcium to contract and magnesium to relax, which is why magnesium deficiency is associated with muscle tightness and cramping. Also, for many years we have known about the relaxing effects of *Epsom salts* baths (Epsom salts is magnesium sulphate/sulphate). To be honest, for many years I believed that Epsom salts were just placebo - that people were just getting relaxed by having a hot bath. Then I read a study that appeared to demonstrate that a large amount of magnesium is absorbed through the skin when we take an Epsom salts bath. This is now known as transdermal magnesium therapy and can be extremely effective in certain situations where oral magnesium is not recommended. There is also a growing minority of health professionals who believe that transdermal therapy is a much more effective way to treat a magnesium deficiency than taking oral supplements.

Originally I thought that magnesium helped anxiety because it aided in physical relaxation. As anyone who suffers anxiety will know, there is a feedback loop that occurs between anxious thoughts and physical sensations of anxiety. By breaking that feedback loop with magnesium, anxiety can dissipate. However, recently research has emerged showing a strong correlation between magnesium levels and serotonin levels. Low magnesium is now clearly linked with low serotonin. Not only this, but a certain study also concluded that for certain patients, magnesium therapy was as effective as antidepressant medication!

New research is showing that magnesium is involved in a range of vital functions in the brain at the cellular level. Importantly, magnesium is a key co-factor in the production of serotonin, along with other vitamins such as folate and B6.

Increasingly, magnesium is being identified as a relatively potent way to maintain serotonin levels – particularly during periods of high stress (which deplete magnesium).

Curcumin

As those who have read any of my other books know, I am crazy about curcumin. This miraculous natural phenolic substance extracted from the popular spice turmeric is being researched for everything from heart disease to Alzheimer's to depression.

Curcumin's effects on the brain are so widespread that I could have included it in several sections of this book, however for the purposes of what this book focuses on, it is curcumin's activity as a MAOI which is of most interest. Curcumin therefore increases levels of serotonin and dopamine in the brain.

However curcumin may also indirectly increase levels of these important neurotransmitters through indirect means also. Curcumin happens to be a powerful anti-inflammatory, which is interesting in that recent research has shown a clear link between inflammation and depression. Depressed brains are often inflamed brains, so cooling things off somewhat is believed to lie behind one of the reasons why curcumin acts as an antidepressant. By normalising the inflammatory process, it is likely that serotonin levels can also normalise, however the link between serotonin and inflammation is still murky. For example, SSRIs also act as anti-inflammatories in some people and this may be one of the reasons they work to treat depression.

Curcumin also indirectly helps normalising serotonin levels by increasing levels of BDNF (brain derived neurotrophic factor), your brain's "fertiliser". Increasing levels of BDNF theoretically accelerates the healing process, which would include your serotonergic system.

Like I said – curcumin is wonderful stuff.

However, just to reiterate (and sorry if I am starting to sound like a broken record), curcumin is appropriate for mild to moderate depression and would most likely be ineffective for more severe cases.

Other herbal alternatives for increasing serotonin

As well as the options listed above, there are also several other natural options for increasing serotonin. I have mentioned this elsewhere previously however it is important to point out that countless plants have biological actions which modulate neurotransmitters. So when you see it mentioned that Plant X or Herb X increases serotonin, it is important to delve deeper to elucidate whether the increase in serotonin is significant enough. This is why St. John's Wort is so widely used – it has a startlingly potent effect on serotonin levels (although still substantially less than even the weakest SSRI, used at typical dosages).

This being the case, there are only a handful of natural substances which have enough serotonergic effect to be considered relevant or useful. On top of those mentioned, there are one or two others which show promise, while needing more research. These include –

Kanna (*Sceletium tortuosum*) – Kanna is an African succulent with a long history of use by shamanistic and ethnobotanist types due to its mind-altering properties. Kanna contains a range of bioactive alkaloids including mesembrine, mesembrenol and tortuosamine which appear to boost levels of serotonin and dopamine. What makes kanna unique is that it is one of the only plant-based sources identified with clear SSRI-like behaviour (e.g. - St. John's Wort appears to be closer to a MAOI, for example). Based on early promise (it has a long history of traditional use, but has only recently begun receiving research attention), Kanna is expected to becoming more widely used by the general population. At the moment, its use is restricted to those in the shaman/ethnobotanical community and those in the know. As with any herbal antidepressants, don't combine with pharmaceutical antidepressants like SSRIs.

5htp – This is the immediate amino acid precursor to serotonin, so makes easy intuitive sense that supplementing the building blocks of serotonin will boost serotonin. Unfortunately, reality doesn't quite match this intuitive appeal, with research studies showing inconclusive results as to whether 5htp could be considered as a genuine natural antidepressant option. However I think this is quite expected when you consider that depression in not only caused by different neurotransmitters (and many people have depression not even "caused" by low levels of neurotransmitters) and even if serotonin is to blame, there can be a range of actual causes. There may be an issue with receptor function, the number of receptors or a range of other serotonin-related problems. If you have an issue with either the precursor to 5htp (the amino acid tryptophan) or the conversion of dietary tryptophan to serotonin, 5htp could be immensely helpful. 5htp is undoubtedly bioactive, as users of the drug MDMA tend to report that 5htp markedly reduces the time it takes to recover, which is unsurprising considering MDMA basically drains your entire supply of serotonin and its precursors. There are anecdotes of people finding 5htp to be the single most effective antidepressant they have used. You could potentially be one of these people, so a trial of 5htp could potentially be an option.

Cognitive & behavioral therapy (CBT)

If you have never received psychotherapy before, you probably imagine a scenario involving old-school psychoanalysis with Freudian questions probing your relationship with your mother, all the while reclining on a sofa while the therapist listens with apparent disinterest. Fortunately this is largely a thing of the past, replaced with modern, scientific therapies like CBT. I am not a trained cognitive behavioral therapist and in any case, there are already plenty of great books available on this topic, written by professional therapists. (Feeling Good: The New Mood Therapy by David Burns is a good place to start.) However, essentially CBT involves the identification and remediation of faulty thinking and behaviour which contributes to depression and anxiety. Have you ever been in a good mood, only to think of something upsetting or stressful, only to see your mood dive? Have you ever noticed how certain behaviours put you in a good mood whereas other behaviours do the opposite? That is essentially the principle which underpins CBT.

Mood disorders like depression are typically associated with distortions in thought patterns ("I am worthless", "I will never feel good again", "If this presentation goes badly it will be a disaster" and so on.) Over time, negative thinking and behaviour will drive down serotonin levels. Only in a minority of cases is depression caused simply by a biological issue like low serotonin. More common, an event or a serious of (usually stressful) events pushes down serotonin levels, with depression resulting. However this misses a key step, which is where CBT comes in. It is not actually the events per se, but the thinking that follows. How would you feel if you left your car in a car park, only to return and find it on fire, a burnt out shell? Pretty bad right? What about if you hated the car and it was insured for more than its current value? As you can see, it is not events per se, but our relationship to them. CBT involves the gradual identification of any thoughts and behaviours which are keeping your mood down or anxiety levels up.

Over time, CBT is associated with the same neurological changes that drug therapy is known for, such as increased hippocampal volume (People with depression often have shrunken hippocampi) and is associated with serotonergic activity normalising. Compared to those who take antidepressants only, people who also received CBT tend to relapse into depression at much lesser rates, suggesting enduring pro-serotonin effects.

Another reason why CBT is powerfully effective at increasing serotonin levels is the subject of the next section.

Sense of Control

There is a very famous rodent experiment that I often tell people about as it is a powerful representation of an important fact regarding serotonin (and general well-being) that most people have never heard of. If you put a mouse in an environment where it receives electric shocks but is able to escape to a safe area or platform, they tend to cope OK. However if you put the same mouse in a situation where it is receiving electric shocks yet has no means of escape, soon the mouse starts exhibiting signs of depression! Post mortem tests on these rodents also show clearly reduce serotonin levels or changes in receptor density.

The human equivalent is the dead end job, the abusive relationship or any other way a person can lose the sense that they are "in control". Many therapists have observed the phenomenon where people can actually handle a large degree of adversity and stress, in general coping adequately. However once someone feels things are out of control or beyond their control, depression and anxiety disorders often result.

The prescription here is clear – Take charge of your life. Particularly regarding things which are affecting your mental well-being. Even sitting down to make a plan on how to rectify your situation will send dopamine and serotonin levels dramatically higher. Go ahead and try it. Identify something in your life that you would like to regain control over. Sit down and write down a plan on how you are going to remedy this situation. I think you will be blown away by the results. In the planning and execution stage, the dopamine boost will be more obvious, however once you have achieved your goal and the dopamine spurt slows down you will find that gradually serotonin levels will rise.

Meditation

So if we clearly understand that stress depletes not only serotonin, but many other key neurotransmitters, surely a logical question to ask is – *What is the opposite to stress?* Surely deep relaxation and a worry-free state will boost serotonin. The good news is that not only does deep relaxation boost serotonin, we have access to possibly the single most powerful relaxation tool and it is completely free (Unless you pay one of those ridiculous places to receive a "special mantra").

Meditation is one of the most powerful brain tonics available, causing a range of powerful *neurotrophic* (the opposite to *neurotoxic*) effects. As usual, my good friend Benjamin Kramer is way ahead of me and has actually written an <u>entire guide to the effects of meditation on the</u> <u>brain</u>. Kramer says –

> *"Researchers reported that meditation also has a huge range of physiological benefits. These benefits include increased cardiac output, muscle relaxation, elevated serotonin and melatonin levels along with noteworthy improvements in chronic pain [10]. Cardiac output refers to the amount of blood pumped by the heart. The more blood being pumped by the heart, the more oxygen and nutrients the body receives. Serotonin is a chemical derived from the amino acid tryptophan which is one of the primary neurotransmitters involved in emotional function (most antidepressants work at least in part by increasing levels of serotonin). Melatonin is a hormone derived from serotonin and secreted by the pineal gland, which produces changes in the skin color of vertebrates, reptiles, and amphibians, and is essential in regulating biorhythms. You may have seen melatonin being sold as a supplement for improving sleep or treating jetlag"*

Even though I am a passionate meditator, I am no meditation teacher and this is no meditation book, so if you are interested, I heartily recommend you check out some of the fantastic books available on Amazon on this very topic. However Benjamin has kindly allowed me to reprint a simple, easy to follow meditation on the breath from his book <u>Brain Renovation</u> –

1. *Sit up in a comfortable position*

2. *Take a few deep, slow breaths and concentrate on the sensation of air passing through your nostrils*

3. *Count "one" on the 'in-breath' and "two" on the 'out-breath' all the way to "10" and then start again at "one".*

4. *When you find your thoughts wandering, just start again at "one". A useful way to notice that your mind has wandered is when you say "eleven" – that's your sign to tell you that you have passed "ten" because you were thinking about something else.*

5. *When your mind wanders (and it WILL wander), just bring it back to "one" and don't get frustrated. This is the number one mistake that beginners make. They think that the purpose of meditation is to completely stop thinking. This is impossible and is not the goal of meditation. The act of realising your mind has wandered and bringing it back to your breath - that is meditation.*

6. *If you do this prior to bed, after a little while you will struggle to stay awake, so just lay down and enjoy the relaxed feeling. You will soon drop off to sleep.*

However I also want to point out that meditation doesn't have the monopoly on relaxation techniques. In fact, if you are currently depressed or suffering from an anxiety disorder, there is a school of thought that says you should avoid meditation and focus on more physical relaxation techniques until you get better. Meditation involves bringing your thoughts into clear focus and for someone agitated or disturbed, this can sometimes be counterproductive. This is where activities such as Tai Chi, Yoga or even gardening can be helpful.

Don't get stuck on a single path up the mountain. Find out what works for you. There are countless relaxation techniques, from biofeedback to binaural beats to progressive muscle relaxation. Don't be afraid to experiment to find the technique that works for you.

Your serotonin with thank you for it!

Loving-kindness

One of the most powerful Buddhist meditation techniques (which has correlates in many other religions including Christianity) is the loving-kindness meditation, which involves filling your mind with loving thoughts directed at those around you, all living creatures and even the entire universe. Naturally there are a range of metaphysical explanations for why exactly this is such a powerful technique for increasing well-being, however from my perspective I am interested in the potent serotonin-boosting effects.

Again, this is easy to verify with a simple experiment. Spend 5-10 minutes thinking about the people you hate, why you hate them (or, if you don't hate anyone, people that annoy you or you dislike). Take a moment to look at your mind-set and physiology. These kinds of thoughts are associated with muscle tension, increased heart rate and *dysphoria* (the opposite of *euphoria*). Now spend the same amount of time thinking about those you love and why you love them. An extremely powerful element of this meditation is thinking about the people you hate or dislike, but trying to view the world from their perspective. Remember, just like you, they were born a small helpless child and have gone through various tough experiences which have shaped how they are today.

Socialise

As I detailed in The Methuselah Project, one of the most powerful predictors of long life is socialisation. Amongst all the longest-lived people in the world, such as those in the small villages of Okinawa, Japan, to their counterparts in Sardinia, Italy, one of the key unifying factors is that they also possess strong community bonds.

As you may have noticed, a key way of looking at serotonin is – *What are the things we do or think when we are depressed? Do the opposite.*

One of the most reliable indicators of depression is isolation. Depression causes people to isolate themselves and isolation in turn, causes depression. And very often, just like sparks and fires, where there is depression, there is often low serotonin lurking. Serotonin is innately linked to home mammals socialise. Alpha male gorillas have high serotonin and submissive gorillas with no power or mating privileges have low serotonin. The human correlate to this is the corporate world with the energetic, resilient CEO and the unhappy bottom-rung drones.

One way to break this vicious cycle is to force yourself to socialise and form stronger bonds with those around you. Reconnect with old friends and distant relatives. Join community groups. Whatever it takes to get you reconnected. You will be astounded at the effects – I promise.

Oh, and if you want to really turbo-charge this process, join a volunteer organisation helping those less fortunate than you. This combines two powerful antidepressants in one – social connection and self-esteem. If helping others was a drug, it would be a blockbuster.

Boosting serotonin is quite simple and logical. Avoid the things that make you feel bad and do the things that make you feel good. Anything relaxing and enjoyable will usually boost serotonin. Massage? Yep. Getting out in the sunshine? Yep. Draw up a list of things you like doing and the things you need to remove from your life. The improvement can be dramatic.

Oh, and one piece of bad news to finish on. This is so important that I wanted to leave you with it. Alcohol is probably the most common serotonin-killer in modern society. Not only does alcohol send serotonin levels lower after the initial high, it keeps you from entering into the deep sleep stage where your serotonin levels are usually replaced. If you think you may have low serotonin, sorry however you will need to either cut it out completely for a while or at least cut back to levels that won't cause you problems.

Dopamine

What is it?

Considering how important dopamine is, our knowledge of exactly what it does in our brains is surprisingly imprecise. As you may have read, dopamine is a *catecholamine* neurotransmitter, which, along with noradrenaline and glutamate, is one of your main *excitatory* neurotransmitters.

You have probably read that dopamine is your "pleasure", "motivation" and "reward" neurotransmitter and that when your brain squirts dopamine it feels great. As usual, reality is a little more complicated.

Our understanding for some time now has been that, when you obtain something important (from an evolutionary perspective) such as food or sexual gratification, your brain releases a pleasurable rush of dopamine to make you feel "good" and thereby encouraging you to repeat the activity. This is why addictive disorders have always been associated with dopaminergic dysfunction, causing people to seek out the same particular thing (such as a drug) over and over. This is considered a dysfunction because it is not hard to imagine the problems that addictive disorders would have created for our distant ancestors.

However recent research published in the journal *Neuron* casts some doubt over this simplified understanding. Joint Spanish and American study found that it is also dopamine that drives you to seek out these rewards in the first place. Not only this, they also found that persistence is likely linked to high dopamine, so the higher the dopamine levels, the more you are likely to soldier on through adversity to achieve a particular goal.

One of the most interesting aspects of dopamine however is how it mediates both psychological motivation (towards a goal or reward) and the actual physical movement which carries you towards whatever the goal happens to be. The part of the brain that is responsible for this, the *basal ganglia*, is largely controlled by dopamine. If you look at a glass of water and decide to pick it up and drink it because you are thirsty, it is dopamine (via the basal ganglia) which controls the initiation of movement which takes your hand to the glass to pick it up. This is why, when the dopamine-producing neurons in a part of the basal ganglia known as the *substantia nigra* are destroyed, Parkinson's disease is similar disorders is the result.

I bet you thought things couldn't get more complicated regarding dopamine right? In recent years the situation has become further clouded by the concept of *reward prediction error*. Scientists conducting rodent experiments have found that the dopaminergic system is even more complicated than we thought. The classical understanding of dopamine is that an animal sees food (or a potential mate) and consequently experiences a pleasurable burst of dopamine to encourage them to see out the reward and then do something similar again in the future.

However there is a problem with this that you may know from personal experience. Imagine you are walking down the street and you notice an ice cream store has opened so you go inside and order the most delicious ice cream you have ever tasted. How good is that feeling? Next time you know that you will need to pass by that ice cream store you will get a little jolt of dopaminergic pleasure thinking about getting one of those great ice creams again. But we all know how this story ends. By the fifth or tenth time (or sooner in some cases), you have grown accustomed to getting that ice cream and you no longer get much pleasure from it. In fact, if you check your mind-state closely, you may find that you *thought* you were getting pleasure but were really just chasing a kind of ephemeral pleasure just out of reach and were simply acting out of habit.

Unfortunately, dopamine is a "MORE MORE MORE!" neurotransmitter and is never happy with the same thing over and over. You need to keep chasing that bigger and better pleasure. Dopamine loves novelty, which is why travel can give us so much pleasure. Put another way, if something (like ice cream) is abundant, the parts of your brain responsible for reward and reinforcement (which use dopamine to signal) lose interest as they assume that they don't need to ensure you take advantage of it because it isn't as rare as first thought.

This understanding underpins the concept of reward prediction error and has thrown up interesting results in animal trials. Researchers found that, when a mouse experienced the same reward more than once, dopamine wasn't just automatically released when the mouse saw the reward again. Dopamine levels only rose if the reward was greater than expected and if the reward was less than expected, dopamine levels dropped.

I call this the *pay rise phenomenon*. If you are expecting a $10,000 pay rise and you only get $5000 you would feel terrible wouldn't you? Your brain (and your dopamine!) doesn't care that a $5000 increase is more than you were previously earning. It only compares your expectation with reality and if reality doesn't match expectation, dopamine levels drop and you feel displeasure.

So, in summary, dopamine likes new things, rare things and pleasant surprises.

The parts of the brain which are chiefly run by dopamine are the basal ganglia (which you already know about), the nucleus accumbens (which is part of the basal ganglia, to be specific) and the ventral tegmental area (VTA). I want to avoid focusing on individual brain structures too much because this is not a neurology book and also when we look at structures of the brain we can disappear down a rabbit hole that doesn't get us any closer to understanding how our mind works. However in some cases, specific mention of particular brain structures can be instructive.

What are the symptoms of low dopamine?

The symptoms of low dopamine are, in general, reasonably unsurprising when you think of it as your energy/mood/pleasure neurotransmitter, however there are one or two symptoms which are less obvious –

Hypersomnia (too much sleep) and difficulty getting out of bed in the morning
By the way, please don't diagnose yourself as having low dopamine based on this alone. Not having a spring in your step when you wake up would probably describe 99% of the adult population! However if this is a chronic problem for you, dopamine may be involved.

Lack of ability to feel pleasure from the things that normally interest you (*anhedonia*)
This is also a tricky one to diagnose because the concept of "pleasure" is ill-defined. In my case, I have come to understand periods where I am anhedonic, but this is only after considerable introspection. In my case, these (brief) periods are characterised by a lack of that excited feeling you get in your tummy when you do something you enjoy or hear good news. It is also difficult to clearly differentiate between "pleasure" and "happiness". Can you tell the difference? This is one of the reasons why people sometimes get confused when they hear both serotonin *and* dopamine referred to as "the feel-good neurotransmitter". In general, serotonin is a more

contented, relaxed kind of positive mood whereas dopamine is a more excited, motivated and (sometimes) euphoric kind of positive mood.

Lack of motivation

For me, this is reflected in less planning of new projects, with more time spent aimlessly surfing the net or watching TV. This does not mean that surfing the net or watching TV means you are low in dopamine. It is more about the mind state that underpins activities like these. If you want to unwind in front of the TV after a long hard day or take a time out to surf the net, it doesn't mean that there is anything wrong. However if you find yourself procrastinating or lacking the spark to work on the projects you normally enjoy, this could be an indication of a dopamine related problem.

Depression

Severely low dopamine can also cause a kind of low motivation/lack of pleasure/apathetic depression. As mentioned in the FAQ, serotonin depression and dopamine depression are distinctly different. I have usually found that dopamine related depression tends to lack the anxiety component that serotonin depression does.

More introverted than usual

Dopamine gives you confidence, so out of character introversion could suggest an issue with this neurotransmitter. However even this point is tricky when trying to differentiate between serotonin related introversion and dopamine related introversion. Low serotonin is associated with a lack of social power (Dominant primates tend to have higher levels of serotonin) which can also manifest with a kind of introversion. Therefore, only use introversion as one of several symptoms to point towards dopamine being a problem as introversion alone is not reliable enough.

Lack of mental energy

Low dopamine can also cause you to mentally fatigue earlier than usual. This lack of mental energy can also manifest via a lack of concentration.

Weight gain

It is unclear why low dopamine is associated with weight gain however I believe it is linked to both the low energy problem and also changes to hormonal signalling. Drugs that boost dopamine (like cocaine and methamphetamine) cause weight loss due to the fact that they keep your motor revving higher and suppress appetite, so logically the opposite must also be true.

Need caffeine to get a boost

Caffeine (among other things) gives your dopamine a modest boost. This is why a coffee lover will get an unusually strong mood boost just thinking about having a cup of coffee. This is also why, under reward prediction error, that second cup of coffee is never as good. For coffee addicts, dopamine hijacks your brain and tells you I MUST GET COFFEE NOW!

Addictive personality

As mentioned earlier, addictions and dopamine go hand in hand. When you become addicted to something, dopamine teams up with glutamate to hijack your brain and tell you that you must keep doing whatever it is you are addicted to. Addictions can include anything related to your reward and pleasure centre (you nucleus accumbens in particular) such as drugs or sex. Addictive behaviour can therefore sometimes be viewed as your brain's attempt to get more dopamine.

Reduced sex drive

Your libido is strongly linked to dopamine. No dopamine – no desire to have sex. There is also a close relationship between dopamine and testosterone, so if you are suffering from low sex drive (whether you are male or female, surprisingly), testosterone could possibly also be the culprit.

How do I increase levels of dopamine?

If you believe that you are suffering from low dopamine and wish to remedy this, there is good news and bad news. The good news is that dopamine is relatively easy to boost via drug and non-drug means. The bad news is that, because dopamine is central to your reward system, increasing dopamine via pharmaceuticals is fraught with addiction risk and tolerance problems. If you discover a way to boost dopamine, your brain will force you, with some degree of urgency, to do whatever is was, over and over. Then, as tolerance takes hold, you will need larger and larger doses to achieve the same effect. This is contrasted with serotonin, which is not typically associated with tolerance and addiction. This is a potential explanation for why methamphetamine (which works mainly on dopamine and noradrenaline) is highly addictive, yet the closely related MDMA (ecstasy), which works predominantly on serotonin and much lesser so on dopamine, is not considered addictive.

My general feeling when it comes to boosting dopamine is to first exhaust all non-drug options before you consider the pharmaceutical route. I believe that dopamine is much more responsive to certain behaviours and thought processes than serotonin is – at least in the short term, as therapies like CBT can, over time, also boost serotonin.

Pharmaceutical options

In general, if you wish to boost dopamine via pharmaceuticals, you are looking at the stimulant class of drugs, as boosting dopamine gives you energy and usually involves a similar rise in noradrenaline. And, assuming you are not suicidal/moronic and have wisely decided to avoid street drugs such as meth and cocaine to achieve this, your options are essentially the two main medications used to treat ADD/ADHD – Methylphenidate (Ritalin) and Dextroamphetamine (Adderall).

Methylphenidate (Ritalin)

Methylphenidate is a dopamine reuptake inhibitor used to treat ADD and ADHD, along with a variety of off-label uses for people suffering from either extreme tiredness (due to narcolepsy or sleep apnoea) or dopamine related depression.

Methylphenidate has always been the subject of considerable controversy due to the fact that it works in a similar way to cocaine, albeit at much lesser potency and addictiveness. Whilst this is technically true, just because one drug works in a similar fashion to an illegal drug, it doesn't make it necessarily "bad". The codeine you take for pain works the same way as heroin. The painkiller tramadol is a serotonin releasing agent just like MDMA (ecstasy).

I boil it down to this – If you are suffering from severe and chronic dopamine related problems, methylphenidate can be a miracle drug that literally saves your life. If your deficiency is more subtle and less disabling, stay away from stimulants and focus on gentler options.

Dextroamphetamine (Adderall)

Your other legal stimulant option is Dextroamphetamine (also known as dexamphetamine or Dexedrine), which is the other main medication used to treat disorders related to attention and focus. While both methylphenidate and dextroamphetamine increase levels of dopamine, the latter is much less targeted on dopamine. Dextroamphetamine essentially triggers the release of your brain's stores of dopamine, norepinephrine and, to a much lesser extent, serotonin.

If you have both low dopamine and low norepinephrine, dextroamphetamine would be a potent option. However if you have a dopamine specific problem or are at the milder end of the spectrum, give dextroamphetamine a miss. Research also appears to indicate that the addiction risk with dextroamphetamine is higher than with methylphenidate.

Nicotine

I have spent a good deal of time recently studying the pharmacology of nicotine, based on an emerging body of research which is painting an altogether more nuanced picture of this much maligned drug. I should point out that my opinion of tobacco and of cigarette smoking remains unchanged. Cigarettes are possibly one of the most evil inventions of man imaginable. According to the World Health Organization, more than 6 million people die each year from smoking-related causes.

However, when we separate nicotine (which is only one of the many bioactive substances found in tobacco) from tobacco, a slightly more nuanced picture emerges.

As part of my research into this drug, I have discovered that there are a large number of people using nicotine patches and gums, despite having never smoked a single cigarette in their life. Why are they doing this?

Nicotine exerts its effects on the brain primarily by activating *nicotinic acetylcholine receptors* (which, I should point out, are named after nicotine, not the other way around). Firstly, this boosts cholinergic neurotransmission, one of the neurochemical foundations required for your brain to learn and retain new information or skills. However, one of the indirect effects of this is increased levels of dopamine. As increased levels of cholinergic and dopaminergic activity are two of the most powerful routes to accelerated brain function, it is not surprising that many have looked towards nicotine as a brain enhancer. Recently, this dopamine-boosting quality possessed by nicotine has even seen it being studied in those with depression caused by low dopamine. Imagine that discussion between the researchers and the potential test subjects! ("You want me to take *what* for depression?").

In the interests of being able to talk from at least some position of experience, for the benefit of you, my trusty reader, I have trialled nicotine gum for a few days. I should point out that I have never ingested nicotine[6], so could be considered nicotine naïve in terms of tolerance. The first time I tried nicotine gum, I neglected to properly read the instructions and chewed the gum like it was normal chewing gum (For those non-smokers out there – nicotine gum is supposed to be chewed briefly before being "parked" in your gums, which slowly absorb the nicotine). Clearly I received a dose of nicotine which was much higher than I had envisaged and promptly became lightheaded, dizzy and a little bit high. Despite this, I can't say that I would describe the experience as unequivocally pleasant, rather, it felt like I was cycling rapidly between pleasant and unpleasant. However this was likely a function of the dose. Subsequent attempts (using the

---

[6] Actually this is not strictly true. Upon reflection, I probably smoked multiple packs of cigarettes passively when I was a child, thanks to the various adults who were considerate enough to smoke in close proximity to me.

correct ingestion method) resulted in an altogether more subtle effect involving slightly increased energy levels.

Unfortunately I have so far been unable to reliably generate either improved mood or substantially improved cognitive abilities. However I should point out that one person (me) isn't statistically significant and also I am not depressed or even low in dopamine (that I know of).

So if I could summarise my experience with nicotine (both practical and theoretical), it would be that it shows great theoretical promise for situations where low dopamine may be an issue, however in my case I haven't really seen enough tangible evidence that would encourage me to consider nicotine as an ongoing option for me personally, as either a learning aid or just a nice "pick me up".

However if there is one key piece of knowledge I have emerged with based on my reading of the research it is that nicotine's addictiveness (something most would consider beyond question) is supported by relatively weak evidence. For example, no sane person would ever question the addictiveness of tobacco, however in trials looking at the addictiveness of pure nicotine, either in humans or animals, there appears to be very little evidence that nicotine is actually the addictive part of tobacco. For example, the pleasant experience felt by cigarette smokers has been linked to substances in tobacco which act as MAOIs – yes the same MAOI action seen in old-school antidepressants.

I should point out however that the topic of nicotine's addictiveness is far from decided, just that there is evidence either way. I am sure many smokers reading this book may point to their inability to eventually give up nicotine patches or gum. However in pure statistical terms, studies looking at this topic have tended to find that nicotine is at best only weakly addictive. I tend to think that different people will respond differently, depending on how they are wired and their environment (stress levels etc.), so the issue of addictiveness should at least be given some consideration by any previous non-smoker considering using nicotine to boost dopamine.

Natural and drug-free ways to boost dopamine

So, would you like to now hear the good news?

Dopamine is amazingly malleable through engaging in particular activities and dopamine-promoting thinking habits. There is a two way relationship between dopamine and your thoughts. Boosting dopamine gives you optimism, energy, motivation and confidence. Likewise, by engaging in motivating or rewarding activities, you boost your dopamine.

There is a fantastic research paper by neuroscientist Kelly Lambert which is essentially unknown outside of very specific scientific circles. This is a shame because this particular paper is fascinating and introduces a novel concept in the field of mood disorders. Lambert puts forward the term *effort-based rewards* to explain the apparent rise in depression across the world as humans have gradually moved away from our traditional, pre-industrial revolution life.

In the distant past, humans had a more direct link between their actions and rewarding outcomes. They would need to bring down a bison or catch rabbits with their own hands. This is a simple reward that your dopamine system is set up for. You do something and it leads to a reward. However now, this has been replaced, in many cases, by a simple trip to your refrigerator to extract food without any effort. Lambert hypothesises that this lack of stereotypical dopamine-promoting activities may be behind many cases of depression across the globe.

So logically, the way to short-circuit this process is to engage in activities (effort) which lead to a rewarding outcome. Have you ever wondered why it feels so great to look at your freshly spring-cleaned house or washed car? That feeling is the concept of effort-based rewards at work. So, if you want to keep dopamine levels high, even if you don't feel like it, do something effortful and difficult which leads to a rewarding outcome. For me, it's writing books. Nothing beats that intense dopamine surge I get when I publish a new book. Your path may be different.

I also believe this is a major reason why CBT is so effective at relieving depression. Not only does CBT boost serotonin, it also boosts dopamine due to the effort-based rewards principle. CBT is very goal-oriented, involving the setting of a range of short and medium term goals as part of your therapy. Setting (and achieving) goals is one of the most powerful ways to boost dopamine that we know of.

So what kinds of activities could this include? In theory, anything that gives you reward for effort will do. So this could be –

Write a book – Of course, I am biased, however have you ever thought about writing a book? With Amazon's KDP program, once you have written your book, all you need is a simple cover and to write a blurb before you can go live across the world. Would seeing your book for sale on Amazon give you a dopamine surge?

Home projects – DIY or renovation projects are perfect activities for increasing dopamine because you can see and enjoy a tangible outcome. There is nothing abstract about a new outdoor BBQ area or a freshly painted house. Dopamine loves this kind of thing!

These are just a couple of ideas. There are literally thousands of different things you could do to boost dopamine in this way.

Interestingly, Lambert also identifies a specific type of activity which appears to be more powerful than anything else – using your hands! Out brain dedicates a disproportionately large amount of area for controlling and sensing (touch) through your hands. Your hands, with their trusty opposable thumbs, are one of the key factors behind the success of humans as a species. So, if you want to really turbo-charge your dopamine levels, create things with your hands. The most obvious ways to use your hands to create is via hobbies like woodworking, knitting, pottery and even making model aeroplanes. However I think that the activity you choose must involve conscious focus on the hands. Mouse clicks won't cut it.

So, thinking about sex triggers dopamine and so does using your hands. Perhaps this explains the second favourite habit of male humans?

In terms of supplements, there are a few options. Firstly, you can try L-tyrosine or L-phenylalanine supplements, which provide the building blocks for dopamine (and noradrenaline). However this will only work if this is the reason why your dopamine is low. For many people, their dopamine levels are low for other reasons, so if you have no problems with consuming enough tyrosine-rich protein or converting tyrosine to dopamine, supplementing with tyrosine or phenylalanine is unlikely to do much. Another option is the herb mucuna pruriens, which contains high levels of L-DOPA, the immediate precursor to dopamine. Mucuna pruriens can be so successful that it is even used by some Parkinson's disease patients to relieve some of the symptoms of the disease.

Another, much weaker, way to increase dopamine is by using a herbal monoamine oxidase inhibitor, such as rhodiola rosea or curcumin, both of which I am very fond of as gentle antidepressants.

Noradrenaline (Norepinephrine)

What is it?

First things first. You may have been confused by the use of the terms *noradrenaline* and *norepinephrine* interchangeably. They are the same thing, however noradrenaline (which is used in most parts of the world) is derived from Latin and norepinephrine (which is used in the USA, thanks to the US National Library of Medicine, for reasons I have never bothered looking up*) is derived from Greek. If you are wondering why I generally stick to noradrenaline, my reasoning is surprisingly prosaic – the word norepinephrine is really, really annoying to touch type. Go ahead[7] – try it!

Also, the difference between adrenaline and noradrenaline is also complicated, however in general, think of noradrenaline as being a neurotransmitter released by and acting on parts of your brain, with adrenaline being distributed around your body to prepare you for "fight or flight".

What does it do?

Noradrenaline is very closely related to dopamine and they are both synthesized by the same amino acid – L-tyrosine. If you stimulate the release of noradrenaline only (and not dopamine), the result is typically just stimulation (rapid heartbeat, increased body temperature, increased alertness). However if you trigger the release of noradrenaline and dopamine at the same, you get a degree of euphoria much more potent than if you released dopamine only. There is a strong synergistic effect when you add in energy to a euphoric brain. This is why pure noradrenaline re-uptake inhibitors (like the ghastly and generally ineffective reboxetine) tend to have a poor ability to improve mood.

However that's not to say that noradrenaline is unrelated to mood whatsoever. Energy can boost mood. However there is a difference between something being euphoric and something improving mood a little. In general though, noradrenaline works better in combination with other neurotransmitters. This is why the older classes of antidepressants (monoamine oxidase inhibitors and tricyclic antidepressants) are actually more effective than the SSRI's (which work primarily on serotonin) common today. However the addition of noradrenaline into the equation is also the main reason these older drugs aren't used any more, as tweaking noradrenaline creates a range of side-effects ranging from annoying (like orthostatic hypotension, where you get dizzy when you stand up) to life-threatening (If you take an overdose of tricyclics like amitriptyline you can actually die, as they are cardiotoxic in higher doses). Fortunately there are some newer drugs like duloxetine and venlafaxine which boost noradrenaline and serotonin but don't create overdose or toxicity risk.

Another way to explain noradrenaline's importance in mood disorders is to think in terms of someone who is depressed and lethargic, with barely enough energy to get out of bed. If you

---

[7] Edit – OK I thought this seemed half-assed so I went and looked it up. Apparently a pharmaceutical company had an adrenaline product called, conveniently, Adrenalin, so it was decided to switch the generic name to avoid confusion. Fun Fact of the day!)

can give noradrenaline a boost, it can act like a jump-start, enabling the person to start recommencing some of the activities that can, in turn, trigger pleasure. However generally, if you give a noradrenaline boost to someone functioning normally, with normal energy levels, there is unlikely to be much boost in mood unless dopamine is also boosted. In actual fact, what is more likely, is that by just boosting noradrenaline you risk triggering anxiety or panic, which is no fun at all.

There is a reason why stimulants used to treat ADHD work so well – Noradrenaline is a powerful modulator of attention. This is not surprising when you think back to our evolutionary past. If your distant ancestors encountered a dangerous animal, it would be fatal if their mind drifted off and started thinking about that lovely cave painting they just finished. Your brain triggers the release of noradrenaline to tell you *"This is really important so you'd better pay attention".*

What are the symptoms of low noradrenaline?

The main symptoms of low noradrenaline are not particularly surprising, considering what it does. They include –

- Lack of energy
- Lack of motivation
- Lack of focus and attention
- Sleeping too much
- Depressed mood

There is a great deal of debate in psychiatry around our focus on serotonin's role in depression. As some researchers have pointed out, if someone presents in a doctor's office complaining of the above symptoms, most of the time they will walk away with a prescription for an SSRI. This is despite the apparent fact that depression caused by problems with serotonin, dopamine and noradrenaline looks quite different. If this describes your experience with your doctor, perhaps it could be a good idea to ask for options that boost noradrenaline also (apart from reboxetine, which is widely considered ineffective) or seek a second opinion.

How do I increase levels of noradrenaline?

Noradrenaline is relatively easy to boost, whether via drug-based or natural options.

Drug-based options

The most potent way to boost noradrenaline quickly is with amphetamines, which probably comes as no surprise. However some other options include –

Tricyclic antidepressants (such as amitriptyline, clomipramine, desipramine etc.) – These drugs tend to act on a wide range of systems in your body and brain, which is why they are often referred to as *dirty* drugs (*clean* drugs tend to have specific actions). However mainly they act as serotonin and noradrenaline re-uptake inhibitors. Each type of tricyclic has differing relative potency regarding serotonin and noradrenaline, ranging from clomipramine which mainly works on serotonin, to desipramine, which mainly works on noradrenaline.

Monoamine oxidase inhibitors (MAOIs) – These older drugs tend to extremely effective, yet comparatively dangerous because particular foods can trigger a hypertensive crisis, leading to death. If you are in a deep, dark hole and are one step away from electro-convulsive therapy (ECT), then MAOIs could be a life-saving option. If you are looking to give your neurochemicals a nice handy boost, don't even think about MAOIs. There is however a key distinction. Some natural substances (such as rhodiola rosea and curcumin) act as weak MAOIs, as does the more recent drug moclobemide. However these are known as *reversible* MAOIs and don't come with the same dangers that the older *irreversible* MAOIs do.

Natural and drug-free options for boosting noradrenaline

In general, anything that increases noradrenaline will be prescription only. The closest thing to a natural noradrenaline booster would be *ma huang*, which contains ephedrine. However ma huang really only increases adrenaline and it is illegal now in most countries.

However behaviorally, it is easy to increase noradrenaline levels temporarily – Just do things that excite you. Looking forward to something enjoyable, with a sense of excited anticipation and then the experience itself will boost levels of noradrenaline.

This is all stuff you should be doing anyway, however I would caution anyone looking to preferentially boost noradrenaline. I always suggest people focus on serotonin and dopamine because, if you get those two right, noradrenaline usually resolves also.

How do I know whether I am depressed (or anxious) due to low serotonin, dopamine or noradrenaline?

It is one thing to regurgitate everything I know on this topic based on the experiences of others, however I wanted to be able to speak with at least some degree of personal experience. So, in the interests of experimentation, I have done something unusual. Through pharmacological means (which I won't go into, as I don't want anyone else "trying this at home" so to speak) I tried deliberately depleting or suppressing levels of serotonin, noradrenaline and dopamine, one by one, to see how distinct the experience was.

The results were quite startling.

First, low serotonin has a very distinct feel to it. In my case, I experienced –

Anxiety – This was the biggest difference between serotonin depressed and dopamine depressed. For me, low dopamine featured a strange absence of any anxiety, whereas low serotonin made me rather anxious.

Lower self-confidence

Digestive problems (For your sake I won't go into specifics, however mostly involved stomach sensitivity and cramps)

Poor sleep quality

Increased irritability (which verged on aggression at times.) Fortunately I didn't do anything silly however felt like snapping at people sometimes when they said something to annoy me. This is very unusual behaviour for me.

Regarding dopamine and noradrenaline I will put them into the same category as it is difficult to target one and not the other. For example, drugs that act on dopamine (such as methylphenidate) also have actions on noradrenaline and drugs that are more noradrenaline-specific (such as dexamphetamine) also act on dopamine to a lesser extent.

In terms of dopamine, the quickest way to send dopamine lower for a few days is via a dopamine agonist, as your brain compensates in the first few days by pulling back dopamine production. For this, I used the restless legs drug pramipexole (*Mirapex*). For me, low dopamine was associated with –

Lack of pleasure

Lack of optimism about future events

Inability to feel excited

More irritable than low serotonin

Waking up in the middle of the night (However this could have been specific to pramipexole)

This experience roughly correlates to what we read in the scientific literature and what we see when patients report their experiences. The main exception was my complete absence of anxiety, which felt rather strange. Whenever I usually get a bit run down or go through a stressful period, I tend to get a little anxious (Stress depletes serotonin). So it felt rather strange to feel a bit low yet experience no anxiety.

However I think it is important to point out that lower dopamine caused by pramipexole is only an issue for the first few days, as with chronic treatment (past say, the first week of start-up) dopaminergic neurotransmission tends to *increase*. Note that I said dopaminergic neurotransmission, not actual dopamine. Pramipexole (and related dopamine agonists such as cabergoline and ropinirole) mimic the action of dopamine at specific receptors (usually D2, D3 and D4). If you suffer from restless legs or have Parkinson's disease, the first few (often unpleasant) few days should never be a factor in deciding whether to continue or initiate treatment.

This information can be used to allow you to get a greater level of clarity around your mind-state before you see a professional who will be able to offer genuine insight into your predicament. Many people see a therapist without a clear idea of their actual mind state, aside from the general feeling that they are depressed or anxious. Knowing whether dopamine is your problem or whether serotonin is the culprit can be crucial as it dictates the type of treatment you may receive. Giving bupropion to someone with low serotonin or an SSRI to someone with dopamine-related problems can be disastrous, so it can be extremely useful to get a degree of clarity around this point.

Endogenous Opioids (Endorphins, Enkephalins and Dinorphines)

What are they?

Endorphins (the word stands for *endogenous morphine*) get all the limelight, however there are two more, lesser-known endogenous opioids – enkephalins and dinorphines. Most people vaguely know that "endorphins are your natural pain killers" (which is true), however most people are unaware of the vital and central role these opioids play in your mental wellbeing – not just your pain sensing (*nociceptive*) system.

The story behind their discovery is a fascinating one. For years scientists knew that inside our brains are receptors perfectly designed for activation by opiates like morphine and codeine. However clearly our brains have not evolved specific receptors with the sole purpose of getting us high on morphine! Most of our brains evolved in parts of the world far from any source of opium poppies. This triggered a mad rush to find the endogenous opioids that these receptors were designed to be activated by. Almost simultaneously, two separate groups of scientists discovered endorphins and enkephalins, which, at the time, was viewed as an incredibly important discovery.

What do they do?

Each of the three main endogenous opioids (I will just refer to them as opioids from now on) activate a different sub-type of the opioid receptor. Endorphins activate the mu-opioid receptor, enkephalins activate the delta-opioid receptor and dinorphines activate the kappa-opioid receptor. There are even sub-types of the opioids themselves. For example there is alpha-endorphin, beta-endorphin and so on. However for the purposes of this book I will just refer to the three main opioids in general terms.

The best way to explain what these opioids do is to use the example of a life threatening injury in our distant ancestor past. Imagine you have just been gored by a sabre-tooth tiger or woolly mammoth (I am not palaeontologist so these are the only two I could think of – I have no idea whether they were even around the same time as man and have no interest in looking it up!). Not only would it be helpful if you had a natural substance your brain secreted to dull the pain, it would also make sense for this substance to calm you down and reduce stress or suffering. This is, in general, what your opioids are for. It is a little known fact that the most direct route to killing stress is to activate opioid receptors. Due to the general hysteria around opiate drugs and their addiction risk, it is rarely ever mentioned what amazing stress-busters these drugs are. If you are stressed out and anxious, your doctor may prescribe a benzodiazepine like alprazolam (Xanax) or diazepam (Valium), however for many people, a small dose of codeine would be a more direct (and less neurotoxic) way to kill stress.

This is perhaps an explanation why some people become hopelessly addicted to strong opiates like heroin, morphine and oxycodone and why others can take painkillers for as long as they have physical pain and then stop without difficultly. Often the difference is the addict has a stressful (either subtly or overtly) existence which is soothed by opiates. However in other cases the addict doesn't have a need to soothe stress, but an inherent dopaminergic issue which creates addictive behaviours. For these people, it is irrelevant whether it is heroin, cocaine or methamphetamine – they are going to become addicted to something.

Another explanation for the appeal of opiates for some people is the theory that some people have dysfunctional opioid systems which are helped by the additional of an opiate drug. For example, some people may not produce enough natural opioids or their receptors may be dysfunctional.

It is also important to point out that your opioid system is closely connected to your other neurotransmitter systems such as serotonin and dopamine. Activating opioid receptors tends to also boost levels of serotonin and dopamine. The best way to think of it is, when you become injured or experience stress, your brain is like a bartender mixing a cocktail of neurotransmitters to sooth the pain and stress, hopefully enabling you to survive, or in the worst case scenario, ensuring you have a comfortable and stress-free death. Everyone's cocktail will have different proportions of serotonin, dopamine, opioids and noradrenaline. Each of these neurotransmitters work synergistically, causing chain reactions amongst each other. For example, brain imaging and post-mortem studies have shown that high serotonin levels tend to go hand in hand with high levels of endorphins.

However opiate drugs have a much stronger dopaminergic component, to the extent that when someone withdraws from heavy opiate use, often by far the worst withdrawal effects are related to the user no longer having their dopamine levels artificially boosted. The worst of these are usually restless legs and longer term, post-acute withdrawal syndrome (or *PAWS*), which involves a lack of ability to feel pleasure (*anhedonia*) caused by low dopaminergic activity.

What are the symptoms of low endorphin levels?

Compared to serotonin, dopamine and noradrenaline, an endorphin deficiency or dysfunction is actually rather rare, in the absence of opiate use. However I believe there may be a key exception to this. I think that adults who experienced chronic or acute stress as a child may be at increased risk of endorphin system dysfunction later in life. As endorphins are key stress-fighters, there is a chance that someone's endogenous opioid system could become dysfunctional after intense demands are put on it through severe or long-lasting stress.

Probably the single greatest indication of low endorphins or dysfunction is (unsurprisingly) poor tolerance to stress. Someone with poor endorphin responsiveness falls apart at the first sign of emotional stress. This is also seen with long term opiate addict, who find themselves completely unable to deal with any stress if they aren't high on their drug of choice.

Another unsurprisingly symptom of dysfunction would be a low threshold for pain or even hyperalgesia, where you find certain things painful that most people would find to be neutral stimuli (like the example of clothes feeling painful or "scratchy").

In general however, endorphin dysfunction doesn't usually occur in isolation. If you have a problem here, you probably also have an issue with one or more of your monoamines, such as serotonin. Therefore in most cases I think the best option is to address other neurotransmitter imbalances first and endorphins should naturally normalise.

How do I increase levels of endorphins?

Drug-based options

Boosting serotonin makes you love everyone. Boosting dopamine and noradrenaline makes you feel a million dollars. However boosting opioids makes you feel like you have gone to heaven.

However there a few problems with boosting opioids (or more accurately *agonising* opiate receptors) with drugs. Firstly, as with anything that feels good and involves dopamine is going to be addictive for some people. However I should also point out that this is nowhere near as common as most people believe. For example, the only study of its kind found that in patients on long term morphine treatment for pain, only 3% displayed any signs of addiction. Remember, addiction and dependency are two separate things. Anyone on long term opiate therapy will become dependent, which means that if and when the opiates are stopped, the patient will experience withdrawal symptoms. Addiction is an infinitely more complicated beast and typically involves destructive and compulsive usage patterns or dosages which are either much larger than needed for pain management or dosage levels which continually escalate. Personally, I find the idea of doctors withholding pain medication for genuine cases where someone is in considerable chronic pain, over a three in one-hundred chance of addiction, quite ridiculous to be honest. At the opposite end of the scale are doctors who hand out strong opiates like candy, when non-opiate alternatives would be more effective. Hopefully there is a sensible middle ground here.

Secondly, there are some adverse consequences from taking opiates for a long period of time or at high doses, however in comparison to many other drugs (particularly illegal drugs), opiates are relatively benign. An expert in the field once explained it as "There are no health consequences from taking opiates, as long as you are happy being constipated and sterile". Long term opiate users mostly adapt to the problem of constipation through various coping strategies (Hint – it usually involves fibre and water), however there are some hormonal problems associated with opiate use, not the least of which is reduced levels of testosterone. Some opiates also impair immune function, so, whilst this class of drug is relatively benign for the brain and body, it is not without consequence.

In short, opiate drugs should generally be reserved for treating pain or as emergency stress-busters in rare circumstances, not for boosting levels of endogenous opioid activity.

Natural and drug-free options

Now for the good news. For most people, boosting levels of your natural, endogenous opioids is relatively easy.

The most obvious and effective way to do so is via cardiovascular exercise (more on this below). You have probably heard of the runner's high, which is apparently triggered by the release of endorphins in response to the pain of exercise. As a side note, according to Benjamin Kramer, this "high" may not be due only to endorphins. In an experiment, researchers gave test subjects a drug that blocks opioid receptors before they engaged in cardiovascular exercise. Surprisingly, the drug only partially blocked runner's high, suggesting the additional involvement of serotonin, dopamine and noradrenaline in this process.

Another great option is yoga, which has also been shown to trigger the release of endorphins via the painful stretching of your muscles and ligaments. In actual fact anything which is painful will release endorphins. If you want to know exactly what endorphins feel like, remember back to the last time you accidentally stubbed your toe on something. As you may recall, whenever something happens which triggers intense pain, after a second or two your brain will release a flood of endorphins, making you feel almost high for a few seconds longer. However this also points to a problem with focusing on endorphins – they don't really last very long – at least in terms of those brief floods in response to injury. However it is important to maintain the natural hum of various endogenous opioids which is constantly at work in the background. Ask an opiate addict how their body feels if they have gone a long time between doses. Everything hurts. Even the sensation of clothes on their skin can hurt. This gives you an indication on how you would feel with no endorphin activity.

If you would like to support your body's natural production of opioids, you can also support this process nutritionally. However as I have pointed out earlier, ramping up the levels of precursors or substances that support any enzymatic process that creates neurotransmitters and neuro-hormones only helps if this is actually an issue for you. Put another way, mega-dosing on the precursors to endorphins is not going to make you high, as your body will always seek to retain homeostasis.

The amino acid d-phenylalanine is vitally important for endorphin production for two reasons. Firstly, endorphins are comprised of d-phenylalanine and a range of other amino acids and secondly, d-phenylalanine inhibits the degradation process of endorphins, keeping levels higher than they otherwise would have been.

How do I increase levels of serotonin, dopamine, noradrenaline and endorphins at the same time, with one easy fix?

There is one activity which reigns supreme in terms of normalising and optimising neurochemistry – cardiovascular exercise. Everything you read about exercise being healthy is true and this is particularly the case with exercise. The human brain loves exercise.

According to Benjamin Kramer, author of Jump Start - The science of exercise therapy for anxiety & depression -

> *"Study after study has clearly shown that cardiovascular exercise and/or weight training works just as well as antidepressant medication, but with one key advantage - Those subjects who treat their anxiety and depression with exercise tend to stay well, whereas those who treat their depression with medication have a significantly higher relapse rate."*

There are a range of theories as to why exercise is such a powerful booster of neurotransmitters and they all may be at least partially correct. As you have probably surmised, whenever I am trying to work out why the human brain does something, I always find it helpful to think back to our evolutionary past. If we look at exercise, your distant ancestors would have typically used intense cardiovascular exercise for one of two purposes – Either to catch dinner or to escape becoming another creature's dinner. Each of these two activities are central to your survival and therefore, the likelihood that you pass on your genes. In this scenario, each of your neurotransmitters has a vital role to play. Naturally, things are more complicated than this simplification, however for illustrative purposes, you can see the following roles for each of these neurotransmitters –

Serotonin – Reduce anxiety, Increase sense of well-being in the event of mortal injury (note that the way the human brain appears to comfort us as we are about to die doesn't increase the chance of us passing on our genes so in this respect, it remains a mystery in terms of function)

Dopamine – Increase confidence, focus, and energy

Noradrenaline – Increased focus, energy, strength

Endorphins – Reduce stress, sooth pain from injury or fatigue

Your brain loves exercise and it is not simply related to neurochemistry. As Kramer details in his book, exercise triggers a whole host of beneficial processes for your brain. One of the most important is the release of brain-derived neurotrophic factor (BDNF), which acts as a kind of "fertiliser" for the brain, triggering repair and neuronal growth.

If, for whatever reason, you can't engage in cardiovascular exercise, yoga is a great option. In fact, the gentle pain caused by a deep yoga stretch has been shown to powerfully trigger the release of endorphins. I have left some yoga classes feeling like I was on an opiate drug, due to the huge amount of endorphin activity I had triggered.

Other Neurotransmitters and Neuro-hormones

Whilst the focus of this book is on serotonin, dopamine, noradrenaline and endogenous opioids, there are other important neurotransmitters which are worth highlighting.

Gamma Amino Butyric Acid (GABA)

GABA is your brain's most important inhibitory neurotransmitter. Glutamate puts the foot on the accelerator and GABA is the brake. If you are like most people, at least once or twice you have acutely felt the effects of GABA – benzodiazepine sedatives (or benzos, as they are commonly referred to) like Xanax and Valium work by boosting the activity of GABA, leading to reduced anxiety and eventually, sleep.

This is why this class of drug is the most potent treatment (excluding barbiturates, which I won't get started on…) for anxiety possible. If you boost GABA levels enough, it is virtually impossible to feel anxious.

However GABA is associated with the same problems (and more) as dopamine – Boosting GABA quickly develops tolerance and then leads to addictive behaviour. Some people believe benzos to be as addictive as heroin. There is also another major, and more important, downside to boosting GABA with drugs like benzos – They tend to be neurotoxic in higher doses for extended people. If you ever saw someone who has abused benzos for a long period of time you would be shocked. These people are completely fried. This is not a path you want to go down.

Probably the only non-neurotoxic way I know of to boost GABA is via anti-convulsive medications like gabapentin (Neurontin) and pregabalin (Lyrica). In fact, because these drugs can prevent glutamate toxicity (Where glutamate levels are overactive, damaging neurons), there is an argument to suggest that for some people, they are neuroprotective. The key seems to be that these types of drugs don't boost GABA directly. They actually boost GABA by suppressing glutamate. To use the car analogy again, benzos put the foot hard on the brake, whereas drugs like Lyrica slow the car by taking the foot off the accelerator.

In general, like endogenous opioids, I am not really a fan of targeting GABA directly. If you have problems with GABA you almost always have an underlying serotonin issue, as they are very closely interrelated. According to author L. Ciranna in the study *Serotonin as a Modulator of Glutamate- and GABA-Mediated Neurotransmission: Implications in Physiological Functions and in Pathology* (How's that for a mouthful?) in the journal *Current Neuropharmacology*, serotonin *"…exerts a very complex modulatory control over glutamate- and GABA-mediated transmission, involving many subtypes of 5-HT receptors and a large variety of effects."* If you want to fix GABA, you can either start taking a benzo (Not recommended unless you have a severe anxiety disorder) or fix your serotonin signalling through one or more of the various options listed earlier.

Lastly, you may have seen GABA supplements for sale in a health food store. Don't bother. There is very little evidence that oral GABA crosses the blood-brain barrier in any meaningful amounts. GABA is like glutathione in that way – you are better off fixing GABA indirectly.

Glutamate

Now that we have looked at your brain's main "brake", let's move on to the "accelerator".

As glutamate is so abundant and so complicated, I could spend many pages detailing the minutiae of all the various things it does inside your brain. However such an indulgence would be against the spirit of this book which is to keep things to key, interesting points that you can use and apply to your own situation.

There are a range of glutamate receptors, such as the NMDA (*n-methyl d-aspartate*) and AMPA (which stands for, get ready for it, *a-amino-3-hydroxy-5-methyl-4-isoxazolepropionic acid*) receptors. Put simply, your NMDA receptors are involved in a range of functions but are most commonly associated with memory, learning and synaptic plasticity. However this doesn't quite capture the sheer complexity of NMDA receptors. For example, drugs that block (antagonise) NMDA receptors can act as *disassociatives*, such as the street drug PCP (Angel Dust) and the cough suppressant dextromethorphan (Robitussin). This is why some people abuse dextromethorphan by taking large doses (*Robotripping*) or do the same with the horse tranquiliser ketamine. If you block NMDA in sufficiently large doses you will literally lose your grip on reality.

So blocking NMDA receptors must be pretty bad news right? Strangely, no, except perhaps in huge, insane doses. For example, one of the hottest new developments into depression research has been looking at NMDA receptors and their role in depression. There is no prescription drug available which can quickly and effectively treat depression, with one exception. Recently researchers discovered that, if you give ketamine to a depressed person, the depressive symptoms lift almost immediately! This discovery shouldn't be understated as this has been the Holy Grail for some time now. So far this has not translated into a widely available NMDA antagonist antidepressant, however this may change in the near future. Interestingly, in sensible doses, NMDA antagonists actually prevent a type of brain damage known as *glutamatergic excitotoxicity*. In fact, a popular drug for treating Alzheimer's (memantine) helps slow the progression of Alzheimer's, which some researchers believe may be caused by excess glutamate. This is also the reason why the food ingredient monosodium glutamate (MSG) can cause problems for some people (Although this is not as common as most people believe).

AMPA receptors are a little more mysterious but no less important. They are centrally involved in fast synaptic neurotransmission and the process known as long term potentiation (LTP) which underpins learning at the synaptic level. One of the hottest new classes of nootropics, which I covered in detail in my book Brain Hacks, is the AMPAkine class which includes the racetams such as piracetam. Boosting AMPA clearly boosts attention, learning and memory retention.

As you may have guessed, the key to glutamate is dose. A little bit of glutamate is great, a lot of glutamate can be very, very bad. The problem is that there are no really reliable ways to diagnose glutamatergic problems, either high or low. If you are suffering from problems with attention, learning or memory, it can be an option to try a racetam or other AMPAkine and if this fixes things, you have a pretty reliable indicator that your glutamatergic signalling is impaired.

Too much glutamate is even trickier. Clearly you don't want to wait until you have developed Alzheimer's (It is also implicated in Huntington's, MS and ALS by the way) before you take action. As mentioned earlier, GABA keeps glutamate in check, so if you have had long term problems with low serotonin (and therefore, often low GABA), you could perhaps be a candidate for excess glutamate problems (By the way, just because you have had depression or anxiety, it doesn't mean you have increased risk of developing one of these neurodegenerative illnesses). According to *Psychology Today*, "having too much glutamate around is to your neurons rather *like whipping your horse to go and go and go until you kill it..."* If you think excess glutamate may be an issue, pharmaceuticals are by far the most potent option. In particular, pregabalin (Lyrica), which works by suppressing glutamate and memantine, which is a potent NMDA antagonist, are both effective options. In fact, there is a fascinating study which looked at the neuroprotective effects of combining both of these drugs into a single treatment for fibromyalgia. This study clearly demonstrated that this combination slowed or prevented grey matter loss in the brain associated with excess glutamate.

However fortunately there is one potent and effective way of reducing glutamate toxicity – the almost miraculous substance n-acetylcysteine (NAC). NAC does so many amazing things in the body and brain that I dedicated an entire guide to it. It does everything from heal the liver (it is given to patients in ER who have taken an overdose of acetaminophen/paracetamol, preventing complete liver failure and death), to treating psychiatric illnesses such as OCD and bi-polar disorder (Note – it is typically used as an adjunct treatment in combination with medications, so if you are currently taking medications for these kinds of disorders, don't stop taking them to start NAC. A better option is to discuss with your doctor whether the addition of NAC would be helpful in your case). In terms of glutamate, NAC reduces the release of glutamate through a fairly convoluted series of steps in your brain. Combined with the fact that NAC also boosts levels of glutathione (probably the single most important substance in your body for scavenging free radicals and slowing the aging process), it is potentially one of the most potent brain health supplements available.

Acetylcholine

Acetylcholine, like glutamate, is a key neurotransmitter for controlling aspects of arousal and attention, however in a slightly different way. Acetylcholine is actually distributed all throughout your body and brain, where is controls a range of functions such as muscle control and reward behaviour. Acetylcholine is possibly the prototypical neurotransmitter in the classic understanding of a substance that is used to send messages from one part of the brain to another, or to the peripheral nervous system. For example, if you decide to pick up a glass of water, there will be a long chain of acetylcholine signaling where the release of acetylcholine is followed by that acetylcholine binding to their receptors, which triggers more release and so on, down the chain, until it results in a muscular contraction that enable you to pick up that glass of water.

There are two main sub-types of acetylcholine receptors – muscarinic and nicotinic. As you may have guessed, nicotinic receptors are so-called because they are activated by nicotine in tobacco. The activation of the nicotinic receptor by nicotine is not directly related to why people smoke. Activating the nicotinic receptor with nicotine triggers the release of other neurotransmitters including dopamine, which is responsible for the pleasure of smoking. Similarly, muscarinic receptors are named after muscarine, a substance which potently activates them.

It is best to think of acetylcholine as one of the types of electricity your body uses to function. To give you a sense of how important acetylcholine is, many venomous creatures kill prey (and humans) by blocking the animal's acetylcholine system (Anything that blocks this process is known as *anticholinergic*). A lack of cholinergic activity is also associated with Alzheimer's disease, however this link is not proven and attention recently has switched to the Amyloid hypothesis which involves the build-up of plaque in parts of the brain.

As acetylcholine is involved in arousal and muscular activity, anticholinergic drugs tend to be sedating. Many of the older tricyclic antidepressants such as amitriptyline, which tend to knock people out like a light, do so mainly as anticholinergics.

If you experience problems with arousal, attention and other cognitive problems, you could have problems with acetylcholine. Fortunately, you have a range of non-pharmaceutical options available if you want to give acetylcholine a boost. The most potent non-drug option is the racetam class of supplements mentioned earlier. As well as boosting glutamate, they also work by giving your acetylcholine a nice bump. My second favourite option is acetyl-l-carnitine (ALCAR), a form of the amino acid l-carnitine which is able to cross the blood-brain barrier and boost acetylcholine.

While I currently stop short of whole-heartedly recommending nicotine (via gum or patches – never, ever via tobacco), for some people it can be quite helpful for giving both acetylcholine and nicotine a boost simultaneously.

Substance P

Substance P is another important neurotransmitter that barely gets a mention, however for some people it can be the source of their problems, particularly if those problems include poor tolerance to stress and exaggerated pain response. Substance P is a neuropeptide involved in the transmission of pain, sending messages from around your entire body back to your brain, telling it if you are injured or have something you should be aware of. Being pain free is actually a dangerous thing, like the people with the disorder *congenital insensitivity to pain*, who can't feel pain and consequently end up losing limbs or dying before their time.

Because substance P sends pain messages back to your central nervous system, if things go awry or become dysfunctional you can either feel pain that is not related to an actual injury (such as neuropathic pain) or not feel the pain you should, causing potentially serious injuries to stay outside your awareness. However in general, neuropathic pain is really the main problem that can be caused by substance P, as disorders involving suppressed pain response are incredibly rare in this context.

If you suppress substance P, you dull pain, however suppressing substance P is only weakly effective for treating pain associated with actual, physical problems (such as inflammation or osteoarthritis). Probably the most common substance P related disorder is fibromyalgia, which is associated with widespread pain that is neuropathic in origin. However it is still unclear whether fibromyalgia is caused by or causes increased levels of substance P.

As we saw in the section on endogenous opioids, pain and stress are innately linked and we see a similar situation with substance P. The best way to think of substance P and its relationship to both pain and stress, let's again cue up the wavy music and gaze back into our ancestral past. Chances are, if you were injured, you were also in a stressful situation that required fine-tuned senses and increased arousal to get you out of trouble. Or, to go back the other direction, if you were experiencing severe stress, it is likely that bodily harm was either a risk or imminent, so substance P levels get ramped up to put your senses on full alert. However, transfer this system to modern-day man with severe stress often unrelated to physical harm, it sets us up for chronically elevated substance P levels, leading to pain-related conditions. Substance P is not raised during mild stress. It only really starts peaking when stress levels are severe or chronic.

Understandably, because substance P is part of your danger-sensing apparatus, chronically elevated levels are associated with sleep disorders and possibly anxiety or depression.

If you want to see substance P in action, just rub some hot chili on your skin. Feel that burning sensation even though your skin is not burning? That is the capsaicin in chilies triggering the release of substance P. However this also points to an interesting property of these kinds of "hot" foods like chili and cayenne pepper. If you consume them regularly, in decent doses, you gradually deplete substance P and this can help improve some pain conditions like the various neuralgias. Cayenne pepper is also available as a supplement which can be effective for bringing down substance P levels. Another surprising ingredient for gently bringing down substance P levels is ginger, so if you suffer from neuropathic pain and have problems with digestion, ginger supplements (or reasonable doses of fresh ginger) could be a no-brainer.

In terms of pharmaceuticals, the only commonly available medication that brings down substance P that I know of is our old friend pregabalin (Lyrica – yes this medication does a lot of different things in the body and brain).

Conclusion

Like it or not, much of our conscious experience is dictated by our neurochemistry. Have you ever paused to think how, one minute someone can view their life as worthless or have a poor self-image, only to take a drug such as cocaine or heroin and immediately have a completely different perspective?[8] Or one minute be in mental and physical pain, take an opiate drug (which doesn't do anything to the actual cause of the pain itself, and suddenly you are in heaven. Neurochemicals are powerful little things.

The problem however, is if we focus too much on neurochemicals alone. That spurt of dopamine is your reward (or anticipation of a reward) for something tangible like an achievement of some sorts, focusing on the dopamine alone is like focusing only on the reward and not on the path that will get you to your reward.

I have always found that the best strategy is to put in place whatever you need to in order to normalise any neurochemical issue (medication, lifestyle changes etc.) and then focus on getting on with enjoying a normal life that is in accordance with the principles of neurochemical optimisation. Obsessing too much over your neurochemicals is a sure-fire way to unhappiness. Your efforts to boost particular neurotransmitters should be treated like an investment. Spend plenty of time initially working out what your issue is and how to address it, then put it away in the bank and get on with life.

Another problem with obsessing over neurochemistry is that, if you reduce everything to neurochemicals, it can take some of the magic out of life. There is nothing I dislike more than scientists desperately trying to explain near-death experiences in terms of neurochemistry. This actually achieves nothing except test the faith of those trying to be strong when faced with their own mortality. If their faith gives them comfort, leave them the hell alone with neurochemical reductionist talk that helps no one. Same goes for love. It drives me crazy when scientists try to explain love as being purely explainable through neurochemistry like oxytocin and serotonin. Love is more than neurochemistry.

So clearly it is a question of balance. Become informed of exactly how your electric brain works so that you know how to live a life which ensures you have the perfect neurochemistry for joy, love, motivation and strength.

January 2015 Update - What about nicotine?

As promised, I continue to stay abreast of the latest research into brain and body health. There are a few things I am investigating which will be included into this book in due course once I have been able to obtain further confirmation or additional analysis of clinical trial data.

However the single biggest update I have is regarding one of the most hated (and, it should be said, loved) drugs on the face of the planet – nicotine. Now, before you take your e-reader and

---

[8] Note that I am not for one minute suggest you do this. You will just feel even more worthless and hopeless when you come down!

hurl it across the room in disgust, hear me out. As someone who has witnessed the horror (and death too, unfortunately) of tobacco smoking, I was surprised to read some emerging research on nicotine. Recently, an expert whose opinion I value greatly said something that caught my ear. He mentioned that nicotine itself is actually an interesting and relatively benign drug – it's the delivery method (cigarettes) that "sucks" (his words). So, as someone with an unashamedly biased view against nicotine, I set about attempting to discern fact from fiction – and what I found was genuinely surprising. Nicotine (like most drugs, including caffeine, for example) is far from being completely harmless, with addiction risk remaining a factor even if it is determined to be beneficial for the brain. However it may surprise you to note that even nicotine's addictive qualities are being questioned, with many researchers now believing that much of tobacco's addictiveness comes from other substances found in the plant.

As nicotine's primary benefits are cognitive in nature (with the most noticeable effects being on concentration levels), I have covered this topic in more detail in Brain 3.0. However nicotine also appears to be a moderately potent way to boost dopamine. As I mention regularly, anything which boosts dopamine naturally creates an addictive quality, as dopamine is the neurochemical of reward and reinforcement. Whatever addictive qualities nicotine possesses will most likely occur through this pathway.

I cover this in the section on dopamine.

I want to stress that nothing in this book should constitute specific advice. It would be foolhardy for anyone to take advice from an eBook, just as it would be equally foolhardy for any author to think that they can give "one size fits all" advice to their readers. This is particularly the case for drugs with potential addiction risks including nicotine or ADHD drugs such as methylphenidate or dextroamphetamine. Any decision you or your doctor makes needs to be a *net* benefit for you. For example, for someone experiencing severe mood problems such as depression or anxiety, any risks or potential drug side-effects may seem small in comparison to the upside. On the other hand, the idea of taking powerful or addictive drugs to give yourself a little boost (or any other subtle desired effects) would seem ill-advised.

Part 3 - Brain Hacks and Nootropics

Introduction

After completing Brain 2.0 and Chill Pills & Mood Food, I realised that together, they formed an unbeatable guide to repairing a broken brain, leading to massive boosts in cognitive abilities, better moods and less anxiety.

However, if we are to target a holistic approach to building the best brain possible, we are missing what I believe to be one of the single greatest methods for constructing a super-brain – exercise. A mixture of cardiovascular and strength (weights) training is one of the most powerful stimulators of brain repair and brain optimisation available.

There is a powerful interrelationship between cognitive abilities, mood and exercise. They are like a tripod with three legs. For example, a completely sedentary lifestyle with no cardiovascular exercise will be tough to negate with even the most powerful of nootropics or mood-boosting supplements. Or, to look at another leg of the tripod, conditions such as major depression or anxiety disorders are associated with brain-fog and cognitive decline. In fact, as you will read later, depression can often lead to dramatic shrinking in the hippocampus – the part of your brain that is central to memory recall. This kind of cognitive decline will be tough to fight with nootropics alone.

For clear understanding, this section is divided into each of these "legs" of our mental health tripod. Proactively tackle all three (as required) and you have the foundation for our much sought after super-brain.

Also, there are a few supplements that have such wide-ranging and potent effects on both mood and cognition that they could have easily have gone in both sections. They include –

- Curcumin
- Omega 3 Fatty Acids
- Vitamin D
- Curcumin
- Astaxanthin

Due to the fact that all three tackle multiple aspects of brain health, I recommend that they form a compulsory part of your supplementation regime. The only slight exception is Vitamin D. If you already get sufficient sun exposure (more than 20 minutes a day of direct sun on the skin, in a warm climate), then usually vitamin D supplementation is not required – especially if you also eat plenty of vitamin D-rich eggs. But hey, you are looking to build a super-brain so I am guessing that you are already planning to eat plenty of eggs right?

Repair and Super-Charge Your Brain with Nootropics

One of the hottest areas of supplement research in recent times has been in the field of nootropics. Nootropics are a class of supplements and drugs which work, via various mechanisms, to improve various aspects of cognitive function such as speed of thought, memory and mood. Some of the early substances which emerged have now become relatively mainstream, including - gingko biloba, brahmi (bacopa monnieri) and even omega 3 fatty acid (fish oil) tablets.

Gradually, nootropic supplements are moving from the underground to the mainstream, with some famous high performers, such as Tim Ferriss (author of the "Four Week..." series) and several high profile venture capitalists/tech entrepreneurs. Famed futurist Ray Kurzweil, known for a dazzling array of inventions and a stack of PhDs, is a passionate believer in the power of nootropics for preserving brain function as he ages. Nootropics are even getting coverage in CNN, with their piece _Are smart drugs driving Silicon Valley?_. Startups in Silicon Valley marketing nootropics are popping up almost on a daily basis, showing a growing demand for cognitive-enhancing supplements. For example, the company Nootrobox has a subscription-based service where they will deliver nootropics to your door each month. Indeed, the company ran a successful crowd-funding campaign known as ""Declaring War On Adderall" to create a safe, legal alternative to the popular ADHD drug.

This is instructive regarding the evolution of nootropics in recent years. Until recently, stimulants such as dextroamphetamine (Adderall) and methylphenidate (Ritalin) were the go-to option for students wanting to maintain focus and mental endurance throughout their long hours of study. Some studies have found that as many as one in four students either regularly use or have at one point used, these stimulants to help study. Unfortunately (or fortunately, if you are out partying at a rave) stimulants like these provide a massive boost to dopamine levels, making you feel food and putting you in a good mood. Anything that boosts dopamine (particularly if it boosts dopamine in your reward centres – the nucleus accumbens and the ventral tegmental area) tends to be inherently addictive. In general I tend to believe that the addictiveness of many drugs is overstated (just about anyone you speak to who has been forced to take morphine in hospital due to severe pain will tell you that eventually they hated morphine and couldn't wait to get off it). However, as you would know from everything you hear about methamphetamines (meth), this class of drug laser targets your reward centres, creating (often seriously dangerous and potent, in the case of meth) addiction risk.

So the challenge has been to find compounds with the cognitive enhancing abilities of stimulant medications but without the addictiveness. For example, if we look at dopamine in isolation, the part of the brain that triggers addiction when a substance boosts levels of this neurotransmitter is different than the part of the brain where dopamine helps boost cognitive functions. When doing your own research, if a substance increases dopamine (or increases dopaminergic functioning) in the prefrontal cortex, you are on the right track. And as I have mentioned previously, dopamine is not the only game in town in terms of boosting brain function.

This is why acetylcholine is arguably the favourite target of researchers in the field of nootropics. Not only does boosting acetylcholine trigger improved brain function metrics directly, depending on the substance, acetylcholine can trigger a downstream boost in dopamine. This is how nicotine works. As I have mentioned before, it is debatable whether this factor alone accounts for the addictiveness of tobacco, as tobacco also acts as an MAO-B inhibitor, preventing the breakdown of dopamine.

Nootropic substances are not just confined to supplements - there are also quite a few drugs available which enhance brain function in various ways. In the recent Bradley Cooper movie Limitless, the protagonist gets access to an experimental new drug which gives him almost super-human cognitive functions. If you are hoping that such a drug exists, well unfortunately I will have to burst your bubble. However there are drugs which are quite similar, if not as dramatic in their effects. I will get to these later in this guide.

The purpose of this section is to distil all the information buried in research studies on PubMed (where scientific studies are published) and break the information down into key points which are easy to refer back to. This is particularly the case for nootropics as they are relatively new as a class, meaning a comparative lack of quality information is available on the topic. Due to the time lag involved, there are powerful supplements, such as racetams for example, which most people have never even heard of. Consequently, the section on racetams alone took quite a bit of work on my part to pull all the small bits of information together into a cohesive single reference point.

Also, for this section (and in general with my books) I have been careful to stick to supplements and drugs with solid scientific backing. This guide is by no means meant to serve as a comprehensive reference for every possible nootropic out there. This is a hand-picked selection of what I believe to be the most effective nootropics and some basic information on some others which may be beneficial depending on the individual.

Also, anyone familiar with neurology and pharmacology will have to forgive any gross oversimplifications. There are no shortage of tomes dedicated to the minutiae of pharmacology and the brain which are impossible to understand for those not formally trained. The goal of this section is to successfully translate that information via simplified analogies and generalizations to enable others to understand what is often referred to as the most complex structure in the universe – the human brain.

Another point worth making is that I will again cover some of the neurochemicals detailed in the previous section, however in some cases with a slightly different context. Some repetition is unavoidable (and indeed actually desirable, if you want the information to stick).

What exactly is a nootropic substance?

Nootropics are basically supplements and drugs which enhance brain function in some way. In general, all nootropics work by either increasing the supply of oxygen to the brain, the production or supply of the neurotransmitters or by stimulating neuroplastic brain growth. The father of nootropics, Dr. Corneliu E. Giurgea, said that, by definition, nootropics –

- Should enhance learning and memory

- Should protect the brain from injury or damage

- Should improve brain functioning

- Should be relatively safe for the brain and be without serious side-effects

In terms of drugs, currently the most widely used nootropics are the various stimulants used to treat ADHD including methylphenidate and amphetamine. These drugs enhance cognitive function by improving concentration, reducing impulsive behaviour and improving planning skills.

Often, the difference between stimulants and other drugs used to treat diseases such as Parkinson's and Huntington's is vague. In general, all of these drugs work by different means to modulate levels of either dopamine or norepinephrine.

How do nootropics work?

Different nootropics work via different means. For example, gingko appears to work primarily by increasing blood flow to the brain, with all the benefits that increased blood supply brings. However, most nootropics work to improve mental function by modulating key neurotransmitters including acetylcholine, dopamine, norepinephrine and glutamate. Of these, acetylcholine and dopamine are central to most processes that improve cognitive function.

My apologies for going over old ground, however before we go much further I think it is necessary to revisit some of the basic information regarding these neurotransmitters – this time with greater reference to their nootropic characteristics.

What is acetylcholine?

Acetylcholine is your most abundant neurotransmitter, due mainly to the face that it is located not only in the central nervous system (your brain, essentially) by also can be found in the peripheral nervous system (the rest of your body). In the body, acetylcholine is required for muscle activation, including your vital breathing function. To demonstrate how important this neurotransmitter is, certain lethal nerve gases such as sarin (used recently in Syria on innocent women and children) work by impairing the action of acetylcholine. In the brain, acetylcholine works to modulate attention and arousal (meaning physiological, not sexual in this context).

What is dopamine?

Dopamine, along with norepinephrine and glutamate, is one of the brain's key excitatory neurotransmitters. Dopamine is an interesting substance; being involved centrally in staying focused and motivated, along with being vital to the process of moving your body. The movement disorder Parkinson's, involves the death of dopamine producing neurons in the part of the brain responsible for movement.

Put another way, evolution has made it so that dopamine moves you (both physically and mentally) towards goals that are beneficial for your survival.

The way that dopamine achieves this is by giving you a sensation of pleasure in anticipating something rewarding. That little burst of pleasure you feel in anticipation of a delicious meal or 'sexy time' with a potential partner is due to dopamine.

As dopamine helps you focus on your goals, low levels of dopamine can lead to conditions such as ADD and ADHD, where a lack of dopamine (and norepinephrine) leads to an inability to concentrate on certain tasks. Drugs like methylphenidate help alleviate the symptoms of ADD by increasing levels of dopamine (and again norepinephrine to a lesser extent).

What is a nootropic stack?

You will often see reference to a 'nootropic stack' if you are researching particular nootropics. A 'stack' is essentially a combination of various drugs or supplements which are 'stacked' on each other for either synergistic (two supplements together provide special benefits not seen with either supplement alone) or potentiating (one supplement increases the potency of another supplement). To give an example, a common nootropic stack may be -

- Piracetam
- Omega 3 Fatty Acids

- Acetyl I-Carnitine (ALCAR)
- N-Acetylcysteine
- Huperzine-A

How you decide to stack your nootropics will be determined by your particular situation. Just because someone else claims miraculous effects from their particular stack, it doesn't mean the same will apply to you. One person's stack which gives them great focus and energy may make another person overly anxious, so you need to construct your stack carefully and thoughtfully.

Racetams

The current undisputed king of all nootropics is a class of supplements called racetams. This is surprising in as much as the majority of people have never even heard of either racetams or the most popular single example - piracetam. Due to the fact that, of all the various nootropics, racetams have the least amount of available information, I will dedicate a larger proportion of this guide to racetams, compared with other nootropics. It is important to also point out that just because racetams are the most widely used of the "specialist" nootropics, it doesn't necessarily mean that they are the most effective for everybody. Like all nootropics, there is a great deal of variability in how individuals respond to racetams, due to the fact that everybody's neurochemistry and cognitive function is different.

All racetams including piracetam, pramiracetam, aniracetam as well as oxiracetam have a 2-pyrrolidone nucleus comprised of oxygen, nitrogen and hydrogen. Whilst this is the subject of a little controversy, the general consensus is that racetams work by stimulating production of the neurotransmitter acetylcholine and/or by improving the uptake of glutamate by activating AMPA and NDMA receptors.

As acetylcholine and glutamate are central to enhancing neural function, it is not surprising then that racetams can have dramatic effects in terms of improved cognitive function.

Since the discovery of piracetam, there have been many more discovered (or created, depending how you think about it), such as - aniracetam; brivaracetam; coluracetam; dimiracetam; etiracetam; fasoracetam; imuracetam; levetiracetam;

nebracetam; nefiracetam; nicoracetam; oxiracetam; phenylpiracetam; phenotropil; piracetam; pramiracetam; rolipram; rolziracetam; and seletracetam. However, for the majority of people, the only racetams they will be exposed to or be able to purchase will be piracetam, aniracetam, oxiracetam and pramiracetam.

Piracetam

Interestingly, Piracetam is a distant relative of GABA (the neurotransmitter affected by drugs such as benzodiazepines to reduce anxiety) and was originally developed with the intention that it would be a potential treatment for anxiety. However early studies showed that rather than acting as an anxiolytic (anxiety reducing), it appeared to improve cognitive function and protect the brain against certain damage such as that caused by dementia or lack of oxygen. It was soon apparent that the mechanism of action was closely linked to glutamate activity at the NMDA and AMPA glutamate receptors along with modulation of the cholinergic system.

The NMDA receptor is central to your brain's process of learning and adaptation via neural plasticity. If we cast our minds back, we may remember that up until recently, scientists believed that the brain was fixed at birth and could not be altered in structure. However all that changed with the discovery of neurogenesis (the birth of new brain cells) and neural (or neuro) plasticity. Now we know that you can change your brain by repetitive behaviours (a concept harnessed by Cognitive Behavioral Therapy) and by selective modulation of particular brain systems, of which the NMDA receptor is central.

Activating the NMDA receptor also stimulates increased levels of Brain Derived Neurotrophic Factor (BDNF), which has been described as a kind of fertilizer for the brain. The stimulation of BDNF is thought to be one of the reasons why cardiovascular exercise and antidepressant drugs alleviate depression. As a central theme in your own research, anything which is positive for BDNF is usually positive for your brain.

The other means by which we can see how important the NMDA receptor is for learning is when we decrease its activity via drugs known as NMDA receptor antagonists, which includes street drugs PCP and the popular cough-suppressant

Dextromethorphan (Robitussin). NMDA receptor antagonists have a clear effect of reducing memory formation, further reinforcing the evidence showing how vital this particular receptor is for learning.

As well as the above effects on the brain's glutaminergic system, piracetam also has beneficial effects on the cholinergic system by increasing levels of acetylcholine.

Acetylcholine is also vital for cognitive function and memory storage. One of the downsides of the older style antidepressants (such as tricyclics) was the negative effects on the cholinergic system, which impaired thinking and memory for many people taking these drugs. Likewise, we also clearly understand the important role that acetylcholine plays in this area due to the fact that diseases such as Alzheimer's appear to be caused primarily by problems with receptor density (the number of these receptors decreases) along with a decrease in acetylcholine levels in particular parts of the brain. Indeed, newer drugs for Alzheimer's patients focus on addressing this issue in the cholinergic system to restore mental functioning.

Recent research has shown the action of piracetam may be linked to another factor unrelated to acetylcholine. This research has indicated that piracetam may exert its beneficial effects on the brain via its ability to improve the structure of the brain's cell membranes. Piracetam appears to improve the fluidity and permeability (the ability for certain substances to go in and out of the cell), thus improving certain cognitive functions which rely on this smooth transfer between the inside and outside of your brain's cells.

So what should you stack with piracetam to achieve synergies?

One of the most common piracetam-based stacks I suggest to those who use my supplement consulting service is to add Co-enzyme Q10 (CoQ10) and Vitamin E. Many of the nasty side-effects associated with anti- cholesterol drugs (statins) such as Lipitor and Crestor are linked to a depletion of CoQ10. CoQ10 is a vital co-factor for healthy mitochondria, which are your body's cellular powerhouses. Vitamin E is a fat-soluble substance which is heavily involved in maintaining optimum levels of CoQ10 and also acting as an antioxidant itself.

These two substances, when paired with piracetam, which improves the structure of the mitochondrial cell walls, provide a potent nootropic powerhouse in my experience.

As previously mentioned, one of the ways by which piracetam appears to work is by enhancing the brain's cholinergic system. This is done by both increasing the density of acetylcholine receptors in the brain and by increasing circulating levels of acetylcholine. One of my favourite nootropics, Acetyl-L-Carnitine (ALCAR) also works partially by increasing levels of glutamate receptors in the brain. ALCAR appears to work together with piracetam to increase levels of acetylcholine by increasing levels of an important enzyme called choline acetyl transferase.

Another angle to consider is to increase levels of choline in the brain via consumption of certain foods or supplements. You can consume a large amount of foods such as eggs or take choline supplements. However my preference is to take CDP Choline (or Citicoline) or Alpha GPC - both of which have been proven to increase levels of choline in the brain more potently than pure choline supplementation alone.

Like many aspects of nootropics, I believe these effects are most pronounced in those over 50 years of age who may have already begun a certain degree of cognitive decline. Piracetam in combination with ALCAR, CoQ10 and Vitamin E appear to be a potent ally in the fight against the common cognitive aspects of aging.

Apart from being the first racetam discovered, piracetam is by far the most popular nootropic drug used among those 'in the know'. Among all the racetam supplements, piracetam has the largest body of research backing which indicates demonstrable effectiveness for enhancing cognitive function. It works by stimulating the acetylcholine receptor system, thereby causing more of this neurotransmitter to be released in the brain.

Users report clear improvements in various aspects of brain functioning including attention and motivation – effects clearly consistent with its relationship to the brain's acetylcholine system.

In terms of dosage, most use between 1-3 grams per day, however you may need to experiment with dosage to find your own sweet spot.

One more thing to note is that when using piracetam and other racetams, is that it is highly recommended to also add CDP Choline, Alpha GPC or another source of choline due to the additional demands which racetams can put on your cholinergic system.

However, in addition to piracetam, there are also some other options in the racetam class –

Oxiracetam

Oxiracetam is a significantly more potent racetam than piracetam so smaller dosages should be required. As with piracetam, oxiracetam can increase motivation, decrease fatigue and improve various aspects of cognition including logical deduction, spatial memory, grasping abstract concepts and other similar higher level mental functions.

A good recommended starting dosage is between 750-1600mg a day. This can be spread out in intervals of every 6 to hours daily. Since it is water soluble, it can be dissolved into drinking water.

Aniracetam

Aniracetam is a fat-soluble racetam, which means that it is slower to take effect and with a theoretically longer lasting action (interestingly, anecdotal reports have often suggested just the opposite - that aniracetam is shorter-acting than piracetam). In comparison with piracetam, aniracetam has a stronger positive effect on the AMPA receptors, more mood enhancement, better verbal fluency and reduced social anxiety. For these reasons, whilst I haven't seen any specific data, I suspect that serotonin is in some way impacted by aniracetam.

Each user will need to experiment with the dosage. As with all racetams, either too high or too low are equally bad so some experimentation may be required. A good starting point may be between 600-3000mg spread throughout the day.

Note that it has been recommended that you take a choline supplement while taking aniracetam in the event that it causes headaches.

Pramiracetam

Pramiracetam has some very good anecdotal support from users who feel that the effects are similar to ADHD medications such as Ritalin (methylphenidate). It appears to be particularly effective for increasing focus and attention and has consequently been popular with students looking to get an edge heading into exams.

Due to the relative potency, pramiracetam should be initially started at a dosage of between 100mg-1200mg in the morning to prevent any sleep disturbances.

So which racetam for me?

This is a similar question to "Which is the best antidepressant?" which you often see on the internet. As with that scenario, the answer is - it depends on the person. Therefore, you may need to experiment with two or more of the racetams to find the one that is just right for you.

One thing you may want to do is seek out internet forums where the various racetams are discussed and read the individual experiences of the people there.

Remember that there is rarely a particular nootropic which everyone should be taking. Naturally there are some exceptions such as Omega 3 (and even, at a stretch, I could controversially include curcumin in this list), however in general it will depend on your particular circumstances. If you have no issues with cognitive function or acetylcholine levels, I can't see there being much benefit in adding racetams to your nootropic stack.

Omega 3 Fatty Acids

Omega 3, in the form of fish oil or krill oil tablets, along with the consumption of healthy seafood, is the single most important thing you can do for your brain in terms of supplementation. Put simply, the brain is made of Omega 3 - well, large parts of it anyway.

One of the key factors in the quick and efficient transfer of information around your brain is the health of your myelin, which is a fatty sheath that covers your nerves. And yes, you guessed it, your myelin is essentially made of Omega 3. You may have heard what happens when your myelin become diseased - Multiple Sclerosis (MS), which is a debilitating, progressive neurological disorder.

Omega 3 is also vital for another reason - it is a potent anti-inflammatory. In your brain and body, to a certain degree, inflammation is controlled by Omega 6 (which increases inflammation) and Omega 3 (which decreases it). Remember, inflammation is not dangerous in itself - without inflammation your body would not be able to heal certain injuries and fight illness. The problems only emerge when the balance between Omega 3 and Omega 6 gets of out of whack. The theory as to why inflammation today runs rampant in humans is that in the past, our diets were more skewed to Omega 3. However today, with our grain-based diet, we consume far too much Omega 6 and not enough Omega 3. Not only do we consume a large amount of grain, our animals are now also mainly fed grains and oilseeds (corn, wheat, barley, soybean meal) instead of grass, so our meat is also now high in Omega 6.

The single best thing you can do to rectify this is to take a large dose of fish oil or krill oil. Certain research suggests that krill may be better absorbed and it also contains astaxanthin, so if your budget can stretch, I highly recommend krill supplements.

There is a fascinating area of research recently which hypothesizes that depression may be associated with elevated levels of inflammation in the brain. As this is early days, scientists don't yet know whether inflammation causes depression or whether depression causes inflammation, however it is certainly a promising line of inquiry. Due to the fact that many sufferers of depression have indicated that Omega 3 appears to help them, this would make perfect sense.

This also appears to be the case for bipolar disorder (manic depression), which is associated with dramatic mood swings and shifts in perception of reality. Many doctors are now supplementing patients with Omega 3 along with their standard pharmaceutical treatments. I need to stress here that in no circumstances should someone read this and think that they can stop taking their mood-stabilizing medication and switch to fish oil. As you have no idea how you will react, this would be incredibly dangerous. If you are interested in the use of fish oil for bipolar disorder, discuss with your doctor.

My preference is to get your Omega 3 from a wide-range of sources. Omega 3 contains two important substances - DHA and EPA. Each source of Omega 3 has different ratios of these two substances and different levels of absorption by your body. The most common sources of Omega 3 include - Fish Oil, Krill Oil, Cod Liver Oil[9] (which also contains Vitamin D and Vitamin A), Seafood [10](particularly fatty fish), Grass-Fed Beef and Eggs.

---

[9] * Due to the fact that cod liver oil also contains Vitamin A, you should be careful to keep your consumption of this at reasonable levels. In some instances, high levels of Vitamin A can be toxic for humans. More is not always better.

Acetyl L-Carnitine (ALCAR)

As I mentioned previously, ALCAR is a potent supplement for improving mental function - particularly in combination with a racetam. The primary mechanism of action appears to be by optimizing levels of acetylcholine, however it also appears to improve mood and motivation via its positive effects on the brain's dopamine system. It is for this reason that ALCAR has been studied as a potential supplement for reducing some of the debilitating effects of Parkinson's disease. Early studies have been quite promising.

ALCAR also acts as a powerful antioxidant in the brain, repairing damage caused by lifestyle and natural aging. This is likely to be one of the reasons why it has shown great potential as a treatment for Fibromyalgia, a condition associated with accelerated brain aging due to chronic stress (this is the same reason why the anti- dementia drug memantine has been studied as a treatment for fibromyalgia - due to its ability repair damage caused by stress and an overactive glutaminergic system).

ALCAR also demonstrates a great synergistic effect when taken with CoQ10, increasing energy levels via positive effects on your mitochondria. It also appears to enhance neuroplastic healing, as there have been studies showing a beneficial effect for the recovery from strokes, where ALCAR appeared to accelerate brain healing.

Alpha Lipoic Acid (ALA)

Most people have never heard of glutathione, despite the fact that it is your body's 'master antioxidant' which not only repairs free radical damage itself, but also acts to recycle and increase levels of other antioxidants such as Vitamin C and Vitamin E.

The best way to illustrate how important glutathione is for your body, let's use the example of acetaminophen (paracetamol) overdose. When someone takes massive quantities of acetaminophen, their liver runs out of glutathione which it normally uses to detoxify and remove various drugs and toxins from the body. Liver failure and death can often result. That's how important glutathione is.

Unfortunately you cannot take glutathione, however you can increase levels by taking certain supplements and one of the best ways is via Alpha Lipoic Acid (ALA).

ALA does not directly improve cognitive function directly by the same means as other nootropics, but works to repair cellular damage in your brain, preventing some of the declines typically seen with the aging process. Recently, several trials have shown benefit for using ALA to treat conditions such as age related cognitive dysfunction, Alzheimer's and Multiple Sclerosis. ALA is by no means a cure for these diseases, however has shown promise in slowing the progression of these debilitating conditions.

---

[10] ** Be careful to keep your consumption of certain fish that are high in mercury to sensible levels. In general, fish at the top of the food chain such as sharks, tuna or swordfish, are the main offenders you need to be careful of.

The means by which ALA exerts its effects on the brain are predominantly via increased glutathione levels, however this supplement also acts as an anti- inflammatory, providing benefit where there may be excess inflammation in the brain.

Phosphatidylserine (PS)

As we discussed in the section on racetams, the membrane of your cell walls is vitally important for enhanced cognitive function. A healthy cell wall enables smooth and efficient transfer of information between the inside and outside of each cell. One of the major components of the cell wall is a substance called Phosphatidylserine (PS).

Supplementation with PS appears to be particularly beneficial for conditions involving poor concentration and memory, such as ADHD. PS also showed promise in a study looking at its possible use as a treatment for depression. My suspicion is that PS would only be useful to treat depression for a particular subset of the disorder. Remember - depression is not a single illness but a collection of symptoms. Based on the way that PS works, I think it would be useful for depression related to cell wall dysfunction or lack of permeability, along with depression caused by chronically elevated cortisol. As you may know, cortisol is a major hormone associated with the stress response. After a period of protracted, chronic stress, levels of cortisol can be consistently high with depression often resulting, depending on the individual's particular genetic makeup.

N-Acetylcysteine (NAC)

I am such a strong supporter of N-Acetylcysteine (NAC) that I even dedicated an entire guide to it. NAC is on my list of supplements that I believe the majority of people out there would benefit from. The main reason is that, as a way to increase glutathione, NAC is virtually without equal. Remember my example of someone who overdoses on acetaminophen? Guess what they will be given at the hospital? Yep, you guessed it - NAC! Just like ALA, NAC is incredibly beneficial for the brain as a general damage repairer and detoxifier.

In terms of specific disorders, NAC has shown great promise for treating Obsessive Compulsive Disorder (OCD) by decreasing levels of certain neurotransmitters which keep the sufferer's brain locked at 'full speed'. Incredibly, NAC is also garnering interest from scientists as a potential treatment for schizophrenia and bipolar disorder.

Due to the fact that NAC can have quite powerful effects on the brain, you should exercise caution. Anecdotally, I have heard many stories from users who either said it made them feel fantastic or feel worse than they did before. It all comes down to your particular brain state and how NAC works with it. If you start to take NAC and notice you feel worse, discontinue and focus your efforts elsewhere.

Choline, Uridine, Alpha GPC & Citicoline (CDP Choline)

As I mentioned in the section on racetams, I prefer alpha GPC and citicoline over straight choline as a means to provide nootropic effects. Both alpha GPC and citicoline are closely related to choline, however with a slightly different structure which enables them to cross the blood brain barrier and exert positive effects on the brain. This group of supplements is vital to a myriad of different processes in the brain, from the production of acetylcholine to the repair of the cell membrane itself. However each has a slightly different profile.

One of the main unique benefits of citicoline is its ability to increase the density of dopamine receptors in the brain. As previously mentioned, dopamine is central to motivation and focus and dysfunction is implicated in conditions such as ADHD. Studies have shown significant improvements in memory formation and recall for subjects taking citicoline. And perhaps even more promisingly, citicoline has demonstrated the ability to reverse some of the brain damage associated with Alzheimer's disease.

The dopaminergic effects of citicoline also mean it has been used successfully to reduce drug cravings for recovering cocaine addicts. Chronic consumption of large amounts of cocaine can lead to significant dysfunction of the dopamine system, so this is quite promising and provides further evidence for citicoline's beneficial effects on the brain.

Alpha GPC has also shown plenty of promise in trials. Like its relative citicoline, alpha GPC has demonstrated a potent ability to improve memory and cognitive function not only in healthy individuals but also in Alzheimer's sufferers.

All three of these choline-related substances also have beneficial effects on mood due to the fact that they are used by the body to synthesize trimethylglycine (TMG) and s-adenosylmethionine (SAM-e), two substances which are central to maintaining healthy levels of key neurotransmitters such as serotonin, dopamine and norepinephrine. You may have heard of SAM-e due to its use as a natural antidepressant. Unsurprisingly, a study showed a strong link between low levels of choline in the diet and levels of anxiety.

The major dietary source of choline is eggs, which I believe to be one of nature's true 'super foods'. Eggs are a nutritional powerhouse and should form a key component of any non-vegan's diet. Unfortunately, whilst eggs are a great way to maintain healthy levels of choline in your diet, they do not contain enough to be used therapeutically and therefore supplementation may be required. But keep eating those eggs anyway!

This is particularly the case if you are an expectant mother or planning on conceiving soon. A recent study showed a strong correlation between a mother's consumption of choline and the IQ of her child. Now, with many study, we don't know for sure which direction the arrow of causation travels. Does choline directly increase the IQ of children because their mother consumes enough of it, or do intelligent women tend to have more nutritious and healthy diets high in choline?

Choline has also shown the ability to reduce brain damage associated with severe alcoholism. Indeed, many swear that the best possible hangover cure is a big serving of eggs, which are jam packed with choline.

If that wasn't enough, like several of the other nootropics I mention, the above three choline-related supplements increase levels of glutathione and reduce inflammation, thereby provide generalized assistance to healing a damaged and inflamed brain.

Arguably, in recent times, even more popular than the above options is to supplement with the closely related uridine, which is one step earlier in the process of synthesizing CDP Choline inside the body. Uridine is a component of RNA and is associated with relatively similar effects to CDP Choline, showing increased working memory and cognitive processing effects like the others in this group.

Which of these is best for you will often come down to your own individual chemistry.

Inositol

Inositol is a type of sugar which is often sold together with B-Group vitamins or choline, despite the fact that it is unrelated to either. Inositol has gained some attention recently when a trial using high doses showed strong benefit as an antidepressant agent and also as a potential treatment for OCD, bipolar and panic disorder.

Inositol appears to work by enhancing smooth neurotransmission, allowing better flow of the key neurotransmitters involved in mood disorders.

Inositol and choline are often sold together as a single supplement due to the fact that they appear to work synergistically, each increasing the effects of the other.

Vitamin D

I am unashamedly a massive proponent of Vitamin D as I believe the recent hypothesis that our modern obsession with skin cancer means that a large proportion of the population are deficient in this vital steroid hormone (it's not actually a vitamin). Vitamin D is so intricately involved in so many different processed in the body that a deficiency can have wide-ranging implications. This is compounded by another slow development in modern man - the lack of organ meats in our diet. In caveman times, if we killed, say, a bison, nothing would go to waste, with all the organ meats also consumed. The meat that modern man eats does not contain significant levels of vitamin D compared to organ meats (liver etc.), meaning that our diets tend to also be lower in vitamin D in modern times.

As you probably know, you obtain Vitamin D primarily from sun exposure. When UV light hits your skin, it causes a biochemical reaction which produces Vitamin D. You should also be aiming to consume a diet high in vitamin D (that means, yes, you guessed it again, more eggs!) or be consuming vitamin D supplements. Please note, however, that if you consume vitamin D supplements, you should also add vitamin K as, without this, elevated levels of vitamin D can lead to increased calcification of arteries - something you really need to avoid.

The beauty of sun exposure is that your body has an ingenious way of turning off the production of vitamin D when a certain optimum level is reached in the body. This is not the case for Vitamin D supplementation, which needs to be done a little more carefully to avoid toxicity, which, although sometimes overstated as a risk, is still something to consider.

In terms of the brain, one of the strongest effects of vitamin D is as an anti- inflammatory. Vitamin D recently gained a lot of media exposure after a study showed that the incidence of Multiple Sclerosis (MS) increase at higher latitudes (that is, the further away you get from the equator). The hypothesis is that a deficiency in vitamin D in colder, darker countries, can lead to chronic inflammation of the brain which then leads to disease of the brain's myelin sheath. Interestingly, darker skinned people from around the equator have less of an ability to make vitamin D from sun exposure, indicating that over time, due to abundant sunshine, their bodies have not had to work hard enough to get enough vitamin D.

Whilst a clear link hasn't been showed as conclusively as with MS, vitamin D has also been implicated in conditions including autism, Alzheimer's and Parkinson's disease.

Vitamin D is also used to produce various neurotrophins which the brain uses to heal and regenerate.

If you want to replicate caveman's consumption of organ meats but can't handle the taste (don't worry, I'm with you - I can't bear the thought of eating liver!), then cod liver oil supplements could be a good idea as they contain omega 3, vitamin d and vitamin A. Be careful with your dosage though as vitamin A can be toxic in large amounts.

Regarding sun exposure, if you are worried about skin cancer or premature aging, just limit your exposure to 20-30 minutes a day, without sunscreen, and you will get a good dose of vitamin d without increasing your risk of cancer.

Huperzine-A

Another supplement which falls in the category of those that few have heard of is huperzine-A. Huperzine-A has been gaining positive attention from researchers recently as a potential treatment for Alzheimer's due to the fact that, like the drug memantine, it reduces damage caused by too much glutamate activity. Huperzine- A, again similar to memantine, functions as an NMDA receptor antagonist and also increases levels of acetylcholine in the brain. Further increasing its credibility as a powerful nootropic, Huperzine A also increases levels of nerve growth factor

Dimethylethanolamine (DMAE)

DMAE is a precursor to acetylcholine and has therefore been studied as means to increase levels in those who are deficient. Research appears to indicate that DMAE improves various measures of attention and vigilance, leading to its use as a potential treatment for ADD and ADHD.

B-Group Vitamins

This is probably the most boring suggestion in this guide but one you can't leave out. So many of your brain's various functions and reactions requires one of the B- group vitamins that if you are deficient in any of them, optimal neural functioning will be impossible.

As you may know, B vitamins are not a single vitamin but a whole group of vitamins which are grouped together as a class with the major link being the fact that they are water-soluble. Vitamins are usually either fat soluble (vitamin D, vitamin A, vitamin E etc.) or water soluble (vitamin C and B group vitamins) with some rare exceptions such as Alpha Lipoic acid which is both. The reason why it is important to know that B vitamins are water soluble is the fact that this means your body cannot store them and needs to constantly replenish levels through your diet. This is what makes B group vitamins an important supplement as it is difficult to ensure you get the right amount each and every day. Vitamin D is stored in the body so if you go without sunshine for a few days it is no big deal. However if you were to consume no B group vitamins for a few days, you would definitely notice significant mental and cognitive impairment.

Any supplement you can buy which has a mix of different vitamins and other substances to fight stress will always have B group vitamins. This is not only because B vitamins are used to synthesize stress-fighting neurotransmitters, but chronic stress has been shown to deplete levels of certain B group vitamins also. Alcoholism also drains the B-group vitamins. Indeed, you are recommended to take a nice large Mega B when you get home from a big night of drinking. It really should go without saying however I will anyway - alcohol is absolutely horrendous for the brain and if you are reading this guide to super-charge your brain whilst remaining either an alcoholic or a binge drinker, you are wasting your time. Alcohol and super-brains don't mix.

Unless you have a specific condition which requires large amounts of a single B group vitamins, I just recommend you take a single 'multi-B' each day to cover off on your requirements.

Here are the main B-group vitamins -

Thiamine (B1)

Thiamine is vital for healthy brain metabolism and for the production of acetylcholine. As a guide on how important thiamine is for a healthy brain, you only have to look at what happens when the brain is chronically deficient in thiamine - debilitating diseases such as beriberi and Wernicke-Korsakoff syndrome.

Riboflavin (B2)

Riboflavin is vital for synthesizing our old buddy glutathione and should therefore be a priority to ensure you have sufficient amounts in your diet or via supplementation.

Niacin (B3)

A recent study showed that niacin offers a degree of protection against Alzheimer's and other types of age-related cognitive decline syndromes. It has also been used to accelerate the brain's healing after certain types of strokes.

Just like with thiamine, as a guide to what can happen if you are chronically deficient in niacin, just look up the dreaded disease called Pellagra which was caused by diets deficient in niacin.

Pantothenic Acid (B5)

Pantothenic acid is one of the co-factors involved in acetylcholine production and unsurprisingly, research has shown that supplementation can provide tangible benefits for memory recall and concentration.

Pyridoxine (B6)

Pyridoxine is essential for the production of of neurotransmitters such as serotonin, dopamine and noradrenaline. Therefore it comes as no surprise that deficiency of Pyridoxine has been strongly implicated in mood disorders such as depression and anxiety.

Biotin (B7)

Biotin, one of the lesser-known B-group vitamins, is vital for the metabolism of fatty acids in the brain - a process central to optimal brain functioning. Indeed brain cells at an individual level require sufficient levels of biotin, with deficiency potentially leading to seizures. That said, I believe actual biotin deficiency to be exceedingly rare and you would generally obtain enough from your diet.

Folic Acid (B9)

Folic Acid (or folate) is perhaps the most well-known of the B-group vitamins due to the fact that expecting mothers are recommended to take folic acid supplements to prevent neural tube defects in their baby. Folic acid is also vital for the production of serotonin. In fact, a form of folic acid is sometimes prescribed as an adjunct to antidepressant drugs to increase their effectiveness. The reasoning is that folic acid helps more serotonin go into the 'serotonin tank' and antidepressant drugs (typically SSRI class drugs such as fluoxetine, sertraline or escitalopram) act to prevent leakage from the tank (yes, this is gross oversimplification but will suffice as a rough analogy).

One thing to bear in mind is that a certain subset of the population are unable to metabolise folic acid correctly and will require it in the form of L-Methylfolate. If you are suffering from a mood disorder or have been taking an SSRI with little effect, it may be worth trying a trial of L-Methylfolate. If you then feel your mood lifting, it will tell you that you are part of the subset of the population with this folate conversion issue.

Cobalamin (B12)

Whist there are no studies which have been conducted using cobalamin to treat a particular illness, there have been some interesting studies showing associations. Among these was a study showing that a B12 deficiency leads to poor results on cognitive tests and another study showing a linkage between high consumption of B12 and lower incidence of Alzheimer's disease. B12 deficiency, which is extremely common in the vegetarian and vegan population, has also been strongly linked to symptoms of lethargy, poor sleep and general motivational issues.

B12 is poorly absorbed from typical food sources such as red meat, so if you are diagnosed as deficient in B12, you will need to have a course of B12 injections or at the very least, take a separate sublingual B12 (by dissolving the tablet under your tongue, you bypass your usual metabolism which leads to little being absorbed). All vegetarians and vegans should get themselves tested for B12 deficiency, however for typical meat eaters consuming a balanced diet, a clinically diagnosed deficiency is rare. That said, if you are embarking on a program of 'upgrading' your brain with nootropics, you will need a bigger supply of all the B-group vitamins, B12 included.

L-Phenylalanine & L-Tyrosine

As I have mentioned previously, the neurotransmitter dopamine is vital for certain higher cognitive functions such as focus and abstract thought. However more is not always better, as Parkinson's patients would well know. Too little dopamine and you experience depression, lack of motivation, lack of focus and inability to feel pleasure. Too much dopamine and you can start hallucinating. Remember, many of the anti-psychotic drugs used to treat schizophrenia work by reducing levels of dopamine.

However I am really only talking about extremes here. In general, my experience has been that giving your dopamine levels a little boost is usually a powerful way to upgrade your cognitive abilities. Naturally, the various drugs that modulate dopamine are the most powerful way to achieve this, however they come with side-effects. Fortunately there are also supplemental options. Which route you go down will depend on your particular situation. If a lack of dopamine production is behind your lack of focus or motivation, then several amino acids and a powerful Indian herb may help.

Phenylalanine and L-Tyrosine are the amino acid building blocks of dopamine. They are relatively cheap and with few side-effects so definitely worth a shot as your first port of call if you suspect you are low in dopamine. However, one thing to bear in mind is that if you suffer from anxiety, I strongly caution you against using these (or any other dopamine-boosting drug or supplement for that matter). Your brain has a finely tuned balance between dopamine (and its close relative norepinephrine) and serotonin. Serotonin is made from another amino acid called L-Tryptophan (or, if you go one step further in the process, 5-htp). Tryptophan is much scarcer and competes with Tyrosine and Phenylalanine to cross into the brain so if you supplement with these amino acids while already anxious (a state highly correlated with low serotonin), this can exacerbate the situation.

Mucuna Pruriens

The step between Tyrosine/Phenylalanine and Dopamine has a step in between called L-DOPA, which is the substance given to Parkinson's patients to alleviate symptoms. Interestingly, a traditional Indian herb called mucuna pruriens is high in L-DOPA and has also been used with some success to treat Parkinsonian symptoms. Many people swear by the cognitive enhancing effects of mucuna pruriens. I tried it for a while a few years back, but did not see any dramatic results however I tend to be a naturally high dopamine person (and slightly low serotonin as a baseline). More recently I decided to give it another try and perhaps due to the fact that I have become increasingly experienced in sensing changes to my neurochemistry, I have found it more noticeably beneficial. It gives a nice clean energy boost and slight bump in mood.

The other key point worth pointing out is that anything which increases dopamine also tends to increase libido and Mucuna Pruriens has long been used in India as an aphrodisiac. As if you didn't need any more convincing…! So far however, in my case, I have noticed no particular changes in libido.

It should be pointed out that, just like L-DOPA therapy for Parkinson's patients, mucuna needs to be taken with a decarboxylase inhibitor to prevent unwanted catabolism and to enable sufficient concentrations to pass through the blood brain barrier. The best way of killing two birds with one stone is to take mucuna with a great natural decarboxylase inhibitor that is also a great nootropic – EGCG (*epigallocatechin gallate*) extracted from green tea.

Another potential side benefit of mucuna (depending on your physical condition) is that it appears to promote fat loss and muscle gain, hence it is used by many gym junkies for this purpose. The muscle-building potential and libido-boosting effects of mucuna both appear to be linked to its suppression of prolactin, the hormone which is secreted post orgasm, causing you to lose all interest in further sexual activity. Incidentally, the fact that SSRI antidepressants caused reduced libido appears to be due to the boosting effect these drugs have on prolactin.

For some people, mucuna can be a miracle and for others, nothing. Whereas some nootropics have predictable effects across the population, mucuna is highly dependent on the individual.

It is also usually recommended to cycle on and off mucuna, avoiding prolonged periods taking it. Only take it indefinitely under expert supervision.

Theanine

Theanine is the amino acid found primarily in tea which is reportedly responsible for the feeling of relaxed alertness associated with consuming this beverage.

Theanine has some fantastic research behind it, showing that it increases dopamine, improves cognition, reduces feelings of stress and promotes alpha- waves in the brain. Also, like memantine and other similar drugs which are effective for Alzheimer's, theanine also appears to reduce damage caused by an overactive glutamatergic system.

Theanine, like mucuna, has wildly varying reports from users. On Reddit, the reports vary from "this stuff changed my life" to "it did nothing". This could be due to differing batch quality or genetic polymorphisms regarding an individual's COMT (*catechol-O-methyl transferase*) inhibition.

In terms of forms, you can either take capsules or consume reasonably large amounts of high quality green tea like *macha* or shade-grown tea (sunlight triggers the conversion of L-theanine to polyphenols). However it would take at least four reasonably-sized cups of green tea to get a therapeutic dose of L-theanine. One of the benefits of consuming it in green tea is that you also get a synergistic dose of EGCGs and caffeine.

Curcumin

Apart from acting as a general anti-inflammatory and anti-cancer agent, curcumin also possesses some fantastic properties for enhancing cognitive function and brain health. Curcumin does so many beneficial things in so many different parts of the body, my friends are all sick of me talking about it!

A recent study showed clear benefit for treating Alzheimer's patients with curcumin. As well as reducing inflammation, curcumin appears to modulate the beta-amyloid plaque responsible for this disease.

It is the anti-inflammatory aspect which is also behind curcumin's recent rise as a potential future depression treatment. The other day I was listening to the radio in my car when there was an interview with a scientist from a local prestigious hospital here in my hometown. He was invited on the show because they were conducting a study into a new hope for treating depression. Surprise, surprise – turns out it was curcumin! The scientist indicated that they had already seen positive results.

How does curcumin treat depression? This is where it gets interesting as it attacks depression from several different angles. Firstly, it reduces inflammation.

Increasingly, many researchers are starting to believe that inflammation and depression are closely linked. It has long been known that depressed people have higher levels of certain pro-inflammatory biomarkers. We still don't know whether it is causation or correlation however there is a definite link. Curcumin, by reducing inflammation, appears to act as a potent antidepressant.

Secondly, curcumin functions as a MAOI, which, as previously mentioned, inhibits the action of an enzyme which breaks down serotonin, norepinephrine and dopamine in your brain, thereby increasing levels. Traditional pharmaceutical MAOIs were extremely dangerous in overdose or if you consumed certain foods like aged cheese or red wine which could trigger a hypertensive crisis. Fortunately, curcumin is known as a reversible MAOI so doesn't have the same health risks.

Curcumin also increases levels of BDNF, that wonderful brain fertilizer I mentioned before. You may have heard that cardio exercise has been found to be an excellent treatment for depression. One of the reasons for this is thought to be that exercise is a potent stimulator of BDNF levels. In depressed patients, often a smaller hippocampus is seen. The hippocampus, as well as being strongly related to memory and context detection, is strongly implicated in depression also. It is thought that by increasing levels of BDNF, you are helping your brain to 'regrow' after a bout of depression.

EGCG

Epigallocatechin gallate is a catechin found in green tea, among other things. EGCG (and green tea for that matter) is a fascinating substance with a wide number of pharmacological effects in the brain.

EGCG forms part of the nootropic stack used by many biohackers, due largely to the solid body of evidence supporting its effects. For example, a 2012 study found that –

> "EGCG administration was associated with a significant overall increase in alpha, beta and theta activity, also reflected in overall EEG activity, more dominant in midline frontal and central regions, specifically in the frontal gyrus and medial frontal gyrus. In comparison to placebo the EGCG treatment also increased self-rated calmness and reduced self rated stress. This pattern of results suggests that participants in the EGCG condition may have been in a more relaxed and attentive state after consuming EGCG."

EGCG does so many different things, I have little confidence in attributing the nootropic benefits to any one factor. For example, it acts as a potent antioxidant, scavenging free radicals which might cause cellular aging in the brain. It (probably) acts as a COMT inhibitor, hence why I recommend you take it with mucuna to ensure that the L-DOPA gets where it needs to go. It even acts reasonably strongly on the CB1 cannabinoid receptor – hence why I occasionally see posts by desperate stoners wanting to find out how much they should take to get high! Despite how demonized cannabis is, agents which activate the CB1 cannabinoid receptor are associated with a whole range of positive effects (in moderation). EGCG may be a way of achieving this without needing to smoke something (yes, I am aware of hash cookies by the way, eagle-eyed reader!)

Bacopa Monnieri

Bacopa is another nootropic which has emerged from Indian Ayurvedic medicine and is now widely used as a "cutting edge" nootropic. Ayurveda has its fair share of unproven and ineffective "woo woo" stuff, however there are some notable exceptions to this, with herbs like bacopa, ashwagandha and mucuna standing up to modern scientific assessment.

Bacopa has a wide range of pharmacologic activity in the brain. For example, a 2013 review on PubMed found that –

> Current evidence suggests BM acts via the following mechanisms—anti-oxidant neuroprotection (via redox and enzyme induction), acetylcholinesterase inhibition and/or choline acetyltransferase activation, β-amyloid reduction, increased cerebral blood flow, and neurotransmitter modulation (acetylcholine [ACh], 5-hydroxytryptamine [5-HT], dopamine [DA]).

Due to its effects on memory recall, bacopa is often referred (albeit with questionable accuracy) as the "herbal racetam". However both appear to work in relatively different ways.

A bonus benefit of bacopa is that it can also act as a weak anxiolytic for those susceptible to anxiety, however nowhere near the potency required for treating genuine, moderate to severe anxiety disorders. Perhaps for a related reason, some users complain that bacopa makes them a little sleepy

My general takeaway is that bacopa is a relatively mild nootropic with a long history of use so therefore suitable for those unable to tolerate more hardcore nootropics such as racetams or even stimulants.

Sulbutiamine

Sulbutiamine is a synthetic derivative of B1 (thiamine) which was created to enable it to more easily cross the blood brain barrier and directly benefit the brain.

Sulbutiamine has an extremely complex mechanism of action. Firstly, it provides a big hit of thiamine to provide a co-factor in the production of GABA and acetylcholine. Secondly it has some weird/interesting effects on dopamine. It appears to boost dopamine by improving your brain's efficiency for using dopamine for neurotransmission. However it doesn't do this by triggering release of dopamine (like an amphetamine) or blocking the re-uptake (like methylphenidate). There is also reasonable evidence to suggest a similar mechanism increasing glutamatergic activity.

Compared to some of the other supplement-based nootropics mentioned in this book, sulbutiamine is possibly closer to a drug than a supplement and is therefore rather potent stuff. Many users report an almost amphetamine-like boost to energy and mood, however this is anecdotal and not placebo controlled.

Perhaps it is best to consider sulbutiamine as part of the "advanced course" and only to be considered once you are familiar with nootropics, their effects and, most importantly, the safety profile of each.

Semax

Semax is another one which blurs the line between supplement and drug. In Russia where it was developed, it is listed on the government's list of vital medicines, yet in the west it is simply an obscure nootropic "supplement". I think the fact that it was developed at the Institute of Molecular Genetics at the Russian Academy of Sciences in Moscow is a good indicator of its heritage. It was originally developed as a treatment for stroke victims, however researchers soon discovered its cognitive boosting effects.

Semax is distantly related to a key hormone known as ACTH and has a unique mechanism of action. As well as modulating NMDA receptor activity, Semax also appears to modulate activity of a host of other neurotransmitters including serotonin, dopamine, histamine and acetylcholine. The end result is a super-potent boost in activity of BDNF, your brain's "fertilizer" I refer to often. In terms of effect on BDNF, Semax is believed to be significantly more potent than any racetam.

Semax's effects lead to major boosts in all aspects of memory and cognition, along with a mood-boosting effect and what can often be a sizable increase in energy levels. It is therefore considered in a round-a-bout way to be a psychostimulant.

Other Supplement-Based Nootropics

The above list is not conclusive, with countless nootropics available if you look hard enough. However in general the cream rises to the top. Some of the more obscure nootropics are like that for a reason. There are others which are reasonably popular but have questionable efficacy or research backing. Others have questionable long term safety. Some of these, such as forskolin or phenibut, I have elected not to cover as I cannot suggest them with any degree of confidence.

Research Chemicals

Here is where we stray genuinely into the territory of the "serious" nootropics devotee. As well as the commonly available supplements, there are ways of getting access to what are conveniently called research chemicals. Whilst this category of substances were originally considered research chemicals and were only used by research organisations, this nomenclature is (in the context of nootropics available to the average person on the street) used to cloak what is essentially public access to unreleased supplements. Retailers of such supplements can put their hand on their heart and say "hey, we're just supplying substances for research purposes". This allows them to circumvent federal regulations restricting access to the general public.

These substances, which are easily identified due to the fact that they typically have codes instead of actual names, are a mixture of soon to be released supplements and some which may never see the light of day. Throughout my books I stress that the information I provide should never be construed as advice (Hey, I've never met you and certainly don't know what's going on inside that head of yours!) and this is particularly the case where we are talking about underground, research stage nootropics.

That said, there are some with some fantastic positive buzz from within the nootropics community. Some of the more promising of these include –

NSI-189

NSI-189 is famous for its rather spectacular ability to turbo-charge neurogenesis (the generation and growth of neurons) in the hippocampus, the part of your brain central to short term working memory and long term memory. However importantly, the hippocampus is also implicated in depression and one of the main hypotheses of depression is that stress and depression cause reduced hippocampal volume[11]

NSI-189 is currently at Phase 1b stage, treating subjects with depression and if the results are positive, it could see an eventual release as a prescription medication.

---

[11] It should be pointed out that the arrow of causation is a point of debate. Does depression shrink the hippocampus or does stress shrink the hippocampus (cortisol is particularly toxic to hippocampal neurons)?

Meantime it is available from selected vendors for nootropics (sorry, "research") purposes.

PRL-8-53

This is another research chemical gaining underground traction due to its potent memory boosting effects. The mechanism of action is still unclear however it appears to boost acetylcholine and dopamine. Whilst on the surface it shares a similar net effect to nicotine, it doesn't appear to possess any addictive qualities (that we know, based on limited use).

IDRA-21

IDRA-21 is essentially a second generation, super potent ampakine like piracetam. It appears to be particularly effective for accelerating recovery from long term benzodiazepine use. Considering just how neurotoxic benzodiazepines (like Xanax/alprazolam) can be long term (particularly at high doses, which is common long term due to tolerance), this could provide a fantastic option for negating or and repairing any cognitive decline

Pharmaceutical Options

In general, unless you are suffering a particular disorder, I am not a huge fan of using powerful pharmaceuticals to increase cognitive abilities. In general, a slow, gradual repairing of the brain is usually a better long term option. Anyone can get more work done after abusing meth or coke, but this is not only damaging your brain but is a zero-sum game in the long term. Sure you get stuff done tonight but then you're wiped out for however long afterwards. It's a sucker's game. There are, however, a few legal pharmaceutical nootropics with relatively safe profiles that can, in some cases, be helpful. I feel I need to include them in here in the interests of balance and for the minority of people that may need a little extra help at the start to get things rolling. Sometimes all people need is a little kick-start.

Modafinil

If any drug could claim to come close to the mythical drug taken by Brad Cooper's character in Limitless, it would be modafinil. Modafinil appears to have achieved that elusive goal of eliminating all fatigue, improving cognition and being relatively free of side-effects.

Modafinil is predominantly used to treat narcolepsy, however is also gaining attention as a study aid and as a drug to help night shift workers. Its mode of action is quite mysterious still at this stage. Typically, anything used to stimulate, or keep you awake, relies on increasing norepinephrine or dopamine. Modafinil does appear to increase levels of these two neurotransmitters a little, but also seems to have other effects which promote alertness such as being pro-histamine (remember, typical anti-histamines make you sleepy). Therefore, unsurprisingly, the best way to bring a premature conclusion to any modafinil experiment would be to take a potent antihistamine such as promethazine, diphenhydramine or even mirtazapine.

The main downside, apart from an inability to sleep for some, is that modafinil is quite hard to get prescribed (unless you have narcolepsy) and quite expensive.

In the interest of experimentation, I tried modafinil several times and found it surprisingly mild. I felt a little more awake (I tried it on days where I had not slept well) but did not feel drugged at all.

Where things get a touch more grey is the availability of a related compound known as adrafinil. The reasonably easy access of anyone to adrafinil points out one of the challenges facing regulators and health professionals. Modafinil is a fairly highly controlled prescription drug. Adrafinil, by comparison, is available to buy online as a nootropics, without a prescription. Why is this so strange? Amazingly, when you take adrafinil, your body metabolises it into modafinil, but with slightly different pharmacokinetics (half-life etc.). Adrafinil therefore tends to be favoured by the nootropics community who take advantage of this apparent loop-hole.

However, like many of the nootropics in this guide, depending on the country you live in, you may not be able to order certain things over the internet and import into your home country. For example, racetams, noopept and adrafinil are theoretically not permitted for import into Australia. However strangely, many users report receiving their package with a note saying it had been inspected by Customs! Others have had the exact same supplements seized. It appears to depend on the luck of the draw in terms of who inspects your package (double entendre unintended).

Prescription stimulants

The two main prescription stimulants which are used to treat ADHD are methylphenidate (Ritalin) and amphetamine (Adderall) and their various related compounds. If you have ADD or ADHD, these drugs can help you quickly get back to normal (whatever that means in your understanding). However, I think a worthy goal would be to slowly build your brain via the other options in this book to the point where you can slowly withdraw from your stimulant medication. At the end of the day, unfortunately, stimulants such as these are rarely neurotrophic unless you have ADHD. So at the very least, you need to be doing all the other stuff in this guide to negate any consequences of medium to longer-term stimulant use. But I want to stress this point – don't be too dogmatic about it. If you need your medication to function properly, stay on it. Taking or not taking medication is not something to be decided via an eBook. Keep an open dialogue with your doctor. Don't read the scare-mongering on the internet regarding stimulants. Out of all the various forms of amphetamine, it is only methamphetamine which is inherently neurotoxic. However that doesn't mean that these drugs shouldn't be given due respect. It is a fine line between the use of a stimulant for nootropic purposes and full blown amphetamine addiction. Don't go there if you can help it.

If you don't have ADHD or ADD, I don't recommend you try these (unless doctor prescribed for particular conditions) as they come with a host of side-effects and unless you have one of these attention-related disorders, won't be particularly effective. I don't have ADHD and tried methylphenidate a couple of times as an experiment while writing this guide. For me, it just felt like I had drunk a few cups of coffee. But again, I tend to be quite 'high dopamine' so am not the best test subject for these drugs.

Also note that stimulants aren't strictly nootropics, as they have questionable safety profiles taken over the longer term. To use another example, MDMA (ecstasy) is not used (at least not typically, or legally for that matter) as an antidepressant because there are some inherent neurotoxicity concerns and essentially ecstasy robs tomorrow's happiness to feed today's. Whereas an SSRI won't do jack for your mood the day you take it, but should (for most people) lead to a gradual return to some semblance of normalcy. To carry this analogy across, it could be said that for most people, a stimulant robs tomorrow's cognitive function to feed today's. A "real" nootropic however should provide safe, long lasting benefits.

However we don't live in a perfect world and consequently, there is a subset of the population with hypoactivity in certain key brain regions who genuinely benefit from long term stimulant therapy.

Memantine

This is a drug that was developed to treat Alzheimer's and is another example of a drug that will only be helpful if you have a specific brain-related issue. The main reason is that memantine is an NMDA receptor antagonist, a class of drugs which is typically associated with decreases in mental abilities, not increases. The reason why memantine increases cognitive abilities in Alzheimer's patients is that this disorder is related to damage caused by an overactive glutaminergic system. So, by toning down glutaminergic activity in people with this particular issue, cognitive abilities are enhanced. This is further heightened by the fact that memantine also modulates dopamine activity in a positive way for Alzheimer's patients.

However, there are several subsets of the population that should consider memantine.

Fibromyalgia is a chronic pain condition that has been associated with similarly toxic glutaminergic activity as that seen in Alzheimer's patients. A very interesting recent study showed great improvements in cognitive abilities for Fibromyalgia patients who used a combination of memantine with another drug that reduces glutamate levels, pregabalin (Lyrica).

The other subset of the population who could consider memantine are people recovering from drug addiction. Due to memantine's action as an NMDAr (NMDA receptor) antagonist, it appears to have the ability to reset particular receptors which are changed by addiction to particular drugs. In this case, it could be argued that the NMDA antagonism is neuro-protective and cognitive enhancing.

I am actually a big (theoretical) fan of memantine, along with NMDAr antagonists in general, as they appear to have a wide range of therapeutic potential. There are not too many substances which can provide pain relief and almost immediate antidepressant effects. Coupled with this, memantine is able to slow (and even reverse) tolerance to certain drugs, which has some great potential in the area of stimulant use and opioid pain therapy.

However memantine is prescription only and you can expect to get a quizzical look from your doctor if you ask for it, unless you have Alzheimer's. It is also important to note that, as mentioned elsewhere, inhibiting glutamate's activity can, for some, act as an "anti-nootropic" – hence many of the other nootropics mentioned in this book act by boosting glutamate, not inhibiting.

MAO-B Inhibitors

There is an enzyme in your brain called Monoamine Oxidase (MAO) which breaks down various neurotransmitters. The oldest class of antidepressants worked this way. MAO can be broken down into MAO-A which generally breaks down serotonin and MAO-B which breaks down dopamine and norepinephrine.

MAO-B inhibitors therefore have cognitive enhancing effects by increasing levels of dopamine, in particular. The most common of this class of drugs is selegiline, which is often used in combination with L-DOPA for treating Parkinson's disease.

However selegiline also has mood boosting properties and is now approved as a patch for treating depression.

Fortunately there are a variety of natural options which also acts as MAO-A and MAO-B inhibitors. The most common of these include curcumin and rhodiola rosea.

Guanfacine

Guanfacine has been used to treat symptoms of ADHD, however works a little differently to other ADHD drugs as it acts as an alpha adrenal receptor antagonist (like a similar blood-pressure drug – clonidine). Because it tones down the adrenal activity caused by stimulants, it is also used to help kids with ADD or ADHD to calm down enough to get to sleep. Remember, attentional disorders are not all alike and depending on what is causing your own issues, different approaches are required. For example, if your dopamine levels are fine and you take methylphenidate, you can develop motor tics from too much dopamine.

Guanfacine has demonstrated a whole host of interesting effects including - improved working memory, better focus and better blood flow to key areas of the brain.

Tianeptine

Tianeptine is a strange, strange drug, as evidenced by its appearance here in the section on nootropics, along with its appearance in the section on mood and neurochemistry. Tianeptine theoretically acts in the opposite way to SSRIs – it is a selective serotonin re-uptake enhancer. Don't be fooled by uneducated comments on the internet suggesting that this is somehow evidence that serotonin is not involved in depression or that SSRIs are ineffective. Serotonin and dopamine often act as yin and yang, where boosting one can suppress the other. This is why SSRIs can lead to low dopamine states with the according blunted emotions and lack of motivation. This is also why I think tianeptine requires more research as a potential augmenting agent for patients taking SSRIs.

By enhancing the reuptake of serotonin, tianeptine appears to boost dopamine levels, leading to a nootropic, mood-boosting and stimulating effect. The nootropic effect appears to be not solely attributable to dopamine, as it appears to also confer beneficial effects on AMPA and glutamate.

One of the major downsides is that, like just about anything that acutely boosts dopamine, tianeptine can be addictive for some, however it is unclear just how prevalent this is as a proportion of overall use. Some people can use the starting dose indefinitely, whereas others can take it once and start pouring it down their throats in ridiculously large doses.

At the time of writing, tianeptine (or the brand name Stablon) is reasonably widely available to order on the internet. Just check the legalities in your particular country.

Nootropics – putting it all together

As I mentioned in the introduction, exactly which nootropic or combination of nootropics you decide to try depends on what your particular situation is. You will need to do some initial detective work by asking yourself some questions such as –

- *Am I low in motivation?*

- *Am I becoming more forgetful? Do I have a low libido?*

- *Does my thinking lack creativity? Am I anxious or depressed?*

However, once you find a particular combination that works for you, the benefits can be quite dramatic. Whether you are over 50 and wanting to slow age-related cognitive decline or help prevent dementia, or whether you are a student or young professional wanting to get a mental edge over others, then nootropics can offer a lot of benefits for many different people.

Think of it as hacking your basic CPU to make careful and specific tweaks to either fix dysfunction or achieve superior functioning. Or, to put it another way, to become not just normal, but better than normal.

Part 2 – Fix your mood

Part 1 focused primarily on cognition - speed of thought, creativity and memory enhancement (or prevention of loss, as the case may be). However, if we are to take a holistic viewpoint of the brain and mind, this really only covers one piece of the puzzle. For the greater proportion of people, the brain's affective states require more attention, fine tuning and often, medicating. When we say affective states, we are mainly talking about mood and emotions.

According to the American National Institute of Mental Health (NIMH), approximately 26% of adults in the US suffer from some form of diagnosed mental disorder in any given year. This makes mental disorders the number one cause of disability in the country! Of these -

- Approximately 10% of the population has a mood disorder (such as depression) in any given year

- Approximately 3% of the population suffers from bipolar disorder in any given year

- A staggering 40 million Americans (or 18% of the population) suffer from an anxiety disorder such as Obsessive Compulsive Disorder (OCD), Panic Disorder or Generalized Anxiety Disorder.

In terms of the human toll, more than 33,000 people committed suicide in the USA in 2006. This only measures what is measurable. The toll in terms of human suffering is also tragically widespread.

For many years now, the gold-standard in terms of treatment for mood and anxiety disorders has been pharmacotherapy (in the form of antidepressant medication) and Cognitive Behavioral Therapy (CBT). For moderate to severe cases, both of these therapies have been shown to work well for many people.

Meanwhile, at the fringe has been various "natural" therapies which have also been gaining popularity with each passing year. Typically, the people who gravitate towards investigating natural or herbal options for treating their mental disorder have been -

- Those who experienced no relief or reduction in symptoms when they tried antidepressant medication

- Those who experienced relief, but unfortunately suffered a range of intolerable side-effects

- Those with a pre-existing passion for natural therapies or an aversion to pharmaceuticals

All the while, the "natural therapies" camp and the "conventional medicine" camp have been eyeing each other suspiciously from across the room.

In the middle of this are a group of people to which I belong. There is a rapidly emerging group of people with the following general belief principles -

- A combination of CBT and medication is the best course of action for anyone with a moderate to severe case of anxiety or depression. Each of these treatments has their own downside - CBT can be costly and medications have a range of side-effects ranging from mild to debilitating.

- There are a range of natural therapies which have been proven to offer no benefits beyond placebo (such as homeopathy) and as such have given natural therapies a bad reputation in some quarters. I have a close friend who was instructed by their homeopath to cease their antidepressant medication and start a homeopathic concoction. This kind of behavior is the reason why all natural therapies are often lumped in the same category. Some people get better after taking homeopathic medicine due to the power of placebo and feel strongly that placebo couldn't possibly account for such a sudden recovery. I often point out that in some clinical trials, more than 20% of patients who were taking the placebo (i.e. - an inert sugar pill) drop out because of intolerable headaches! If someone's allergies clear up after taking homeopathic medicine, that's fantastic. However pushing homeopathic medication onto a segment of the population that are potential suicide risks is reckless in the extreme.

- There are however, certain herbs, supplements and nutritional therapies which have solid scientific background for treating mild to moderate cases. The lag between clinical trial results being announced and regular use is often quite prolonged. So, for example, despite the amazing results of curcumin in recent clinical trials, you are unlikely to find any doctors recommending it yet for mild depression.

- The single greatest treatment for most forms of anxiety or depression is cardiovascular exercise and resistance (weight) training. In this guide I will be focusing on supplements and nutrition to treat mild to moderate cases of anxiety and depression. I will focus on exercise therapy in a future book which I am currently researching. So keep an eye out for this book once it is finished and published.

As with my other books and guides, the aim of this book is to distil the latest research on natural, drug-free treatments for anxiety and depression into an easy to read reference guide. Most people haven't even heard of curcumin or rhodiola rosea, let alone be aware of the fantastic research which has recently emerged that supports these and other natural therapies.

However, before we proceed, I need to make some important points completely clear -

- If you are currently moderately to severely anxious or depressed, the answer to your troubles does not lie within any book. Please urgently visit your primary care provider to receive professional treatment. The target for this guide is someone who -

- Has been feeling a little below par and possibly mildly depressed

- Has been a little anxious recently or has a long term mildly anxious personality

- Is lacking in spark or motivation

- Was previously depressed, sought treatment and is now looking for non- pharmacological options now that the acute phase has passed. Please note, only come off your medication under the guidance of a trained professional. This guide is not designed to prompt anyone to suddenly stop their medication

- Just because something is "natural", it does not mean that you don't have to accord it due respect. In some cases, the supplements or herbs used to treat mental disorders are surprisingly powerful. For example, St. John's Wort can cause problems if combined with another pharmaceutical antidepressant, due to its powerful effects on your serotonin system.

- Likewise, many supplements interact with each other and with other drugs, potentially causing problems. To use the example of St. John's Wort again, this herb can cause powerful changes in the way that your body metabolises certain drugs, leading to possible complications. If you are planning on starting any natural therapy, get the advice of a trained professional and make sure you clearly mention any other drugs you may be taking.

- Any new exercise regime should also be cleared with your physician, who will take into account your cardiovascular health, joint condition or any other physical issue that may cause safety problems.

"Chill Pills"

I have a confession to make - I am from a scientific background and am not afraid to admit that I have gone full circle on natural therapies for depression. Many years ago I started with initial optimism regarding the first herbal treatments (such   as St. John's Wort) for mental disorders. I thought we had discovered natural alternatives to strong pharmaceuticals which would hopefully lead to less side- effects. However I was quickly turned off this area due to the lack of rigorous studies supporting some of these natural therapies and the lack of efficacy when compared to existing medications. I was also disappointed in the lack of ethical behaviour by many in the 'natural health' field. Everyone is well aware of the often dubious behaviour of 'Big Pharma', so I was disappointed to see that the behaviour on the other side of the fence was often no better.

However, eventually I started to see some really interesting studies emerge which appeared to show good efficacy for certain treatments. Slowly I started to read comments from various people indicating that they found great relief from their anxiety or depression that they were unable to achieve with pharmaceuticals.

Before I look at individual options, I need to make the following points clear to enable a greater understanding of what we are talking about -

- Any "natural" substance which alleviates mental disorders, works roughly identically to pharmaceuticals. Just because something is "natural", it doesn't mean that it necessarily works to alleviate anxiety or depression via magic. In general, anything that treats depression does so by either -

  o Blocking the re-uptake of serotonin - This is how selective serotonin re-uptake inhibitors (such as Prozac, Zoloft or Lexapro) work. Normally your brain removes serotonin from the synapse after it has done its job, however SSRIs block this, leading to more serotonin floating around.

  o Blocking the re-uptake of dopamine and norepinephrine, leading to greater levels

  o Inhibiting the action of monoamine oxidase - These drugs are called monoamine oxidase inhibitors (MAOIs). Monoamine oxidase breaks down monoamines (primarily serotonin, norepinephrine and dopamine), so by stopping this process, more of these neurotransmitters remain in the synapse.

  o Antagonising or agonising serotonin, dopamine or norepinephrine receptors. This either blocks the activity of sub-receptors that worsen

- o anxiety or depression or activating the sub-receptors which improve mood and lessen anxiety
- o Stimulating the repair of your hippocampus - The hippocampi of those suffering from depression are often atrophied (smaller than normal). The regeneration of the hippocampus (via brain plasticity) is associated with an improvement in mental disorders
- o Increasing production of brain-derived neurotrophic factor (BDNF) -
- o BDNF is a kind of brain fertilizer that assists the brain to repair itself
- o Reducing levels of stress hormones and neurotransmitters such as substance P and cortisol.
- o Reducing levels of your brain's primary excitatory neurotransmitter – glutamate.
- o Increasing levels of gamma amino butyric acid (GABA) – your brain's primary calming neurotransmitter. Benzodiazepine drugs such as alprazolam (Xanax) work via this mechanism.

Secondly, just because something is natural, that doesn't make it completely benign and harmless. The various supplements available to help treat mental disorders need to be given due respect. Whilst you can usually dose quite aggressively with natural therapies, that doesn't mean you can pop them in your mouth like Tic-Tacs. Stick roughly to recommended dosages.

Another important point specific to anxiety also should be pointed out. Reducing anxiety (whether by drugs or supplements) is approached from two different angles –

1. Short term – These are substances and drugs taken to reduce anxiety acutely. What I mean by this is that you take something and shortly after you experience a drop in anxiety levels. This is almost always achieved by increasing levels of GABA (via benzodiazepine drugs mainly) or reducing levels of norepinephrine (via beta blocker such as propranolol (Inderal) or adrenal receptor antagonists (such as clonidine (Catapres). There are also a range of potent natural substances which can also achieve this.

2. Medium to longer term – These are the substances which slowly, over time, begin to reduce anxiety – usually by slowly increasing levels of serotonin. There are arguably no supplements or drugs than reduce anxiety acutely by increasing serotonin – with the possible exception of the painkiller tramadol or the party drug MDMA (Ecstasy)

Therefore, the first part of this section on Chill Pills will be focused on reducing depression and anxiety slowly, over time. The second part will focus on supplements which reduce anxiety acutely, reducing levels of physiological arousal quickly, enabling you to calm down and relax.

Before we proceed I should also point out that I will only include substances with strong research backing or experiential data. Naturally this means that (unless new data emerges), I won't be covering anything with poor or unproven efficacy - such as homeopathy or aromatherapy.

This section will focus on supplements which gradually heal your brain to help you overcome depression. Nothing in this section will allow you to suddenly feel "happy" after taking a dose. There are no quick-fixes for healing depression. Any lasting change takes time, so patience is required. As with pharmaceuticals such as SSRIs, you should expect to see some improvements around the 2-3 week mark, followed by genuine recovery starting around the 3 month mark. This magical "3 month" number is not plucked out of thin air. This is the approximate time is takes your brain to making neuroplastic changes such as – improved receptor activity/density or increased hippocampal volume.

Note that I will dedicate most time to the two most potent herbal antidepressants - St. John's Wort and rhodiola rosea. You could also arguably put curcumin into this category at well.

St. John's Wort

St. John's Wort is the undisputed king of herbal antidepressants for good reason.

It potently increases levels of serotonin, has a long history of widespread use (making clinical studies more statistically significant) and is associated with none of the severe side-effects usually associated with pharmacological antidepressants.

Despite the growing popularity of St. John's Wort in the United States, with sales rapidly approaching $1billion per annum, it is far more widely used in Europe, where it turns over more than $7 billion per annum. It is particularly popular in Germany, where there are approximately twenty times more prescriptions written for St. John's Wort than for Prozac (fluoxetine). Amazingly, if you visit your doctor in Germany complaining of mild to moderate depression or anxiety, there is a strong chance you will be prescribed St. John's Wort before an SSRI drug. Now, I always recommend people to be healthily skeptical regarding the efficacy of any treatment, so in the case of St. John's Wort, large sales numbers or prescription volumes does not equal effectiveness and safety as an antidepressant. Therefore part of the purpose of this guide is to outline some of the key research results regarding this extremely interesting herb.

St. John's Wort (or Hypericum perforatum) is a perennial flowering herb native to Europe and some parts of Asia and Africa. It is easily recognised due to its beautiful yellow flowers. Yes, the yellow flowers have nothing to do with how it works as an antidepressant however if you are an avid gardener in the right geography, I highly recommend trying to grow St. John's Wort - it looks amazing in my own garden!

From this point on, as I described the active components of St. John's Wort and the mechanism of action, I will refer to hypericum, rather than St. John's Wort.

Hypericum contains an astounding range of bioactive flavonoids including hyperoside, quercitrin, isoquercitrin, rutin, quercetin, campferol, luteolin and myricetin, along with other compounds such as hyperforin and adhyperforin. However in terms of antidepressant effects, the two main compounds that scientists are interested in are hyperforin and hypericin.

What does the research say?

Hypericum has an impressive body of individual research studies and meta- analyses (where groups of studies are pooled together for better statistical significance) backing its use for mild to moderate depression, including -

- A 1995 meta-analysis of twelve individual trials founds that hypericum was significantly superior to a placebo (an "inert" sugar pill with no active ingredients) and as effective as modern pharmaceuticals at relieving depression

- A 1996 meta-analysis found that hypericum was almost three times more effective than placebo, with an efficacy that matched tricyclic antidepressants for the treatment of mild to moderate depression. Not only this, but hypericum was found to be significantly safer and with much milder side-effects.

- A more recent meta-analysis with stricter criteria was a little more subdued, albeit still with a positive outcome. This trial found that hypericum was 1.5 times as effective as placebo, but also concluded that hypericum was as effective as tricyclic drugs.

- Another study concluded that, while hypericum was effective for

- treating mild to moderate depression, it was slightly less effective than tricyclic drugs.
- A 1999 study found that hypericum was as effective as Prozac (fluoxetine) for the treatment of mild to moderate depression in the elderly.

However it should also be noted that these studies and meta-analyses, like most clinical studies, were not without criticism. One consistently strange result often observed is that the results in Germany are always more positive than the results in other countries. So far, no one has been able to provide a satisfactory answer to why this could be the case. Another piece of criticism is regarding the dosages of the tricyclic drugs used in the trials, which critics have indicated is too low. Critics say that if the doses of tricyclic drugs were increased, there would be a clear advantage over hypericum. This may be the case, however my experience with tricyclics has always been that most people stop using them because of the intolerable side effects (weight gain, constipation, dry mouth, blurred vision, difficulty urinating, dizziness, sleepiness, loss of libido, sexual dysfunction etc.). So if you ramp up the dose of a tricylic you often find people dropping out, making it difficult to assess the efficacy compared to hypericum.

The other major component of hypericum's ability to treat depression is its ability to also concurrently treat the biomarkers of chronic stress. Stress and depression go hand in hand. It is often after a period of unrelenting stress that depression can result. Hypericum has been testing on rodents, where they are given hypericum before being subjected to various stressful situations (as an aside, everyone should take a moment to thank all these poor rodents that suffer so that we might not).

In all the various measurements of stress response, hypericum has been shown to reduce the biomarkers of stress, such as cortisol levels.

Depression and chronic stress is also often associated with disturbances in the HPA (hypothalamus pituitary adrenal) axis, your brain's (and body's) system for dealing with stress. Hypericum has also been shown to positively modulate that HPA axis, leading to amelioration of certain aspects of acute and chronic stress.

That said, based on my assessment of all the clinical literature, there appears to be little doubt that hypericum is an effective antidepressant. However one clear point needs to be made - As with any non-pharmaceutical treatment for depression, hypericum is often a better option than drugs such as SSRIs (selective serotonin re- uptake inhibitors), tricyclics and MAOIs (monoamine oxidase inhibitors) for mild to moderate cases of depression and anxiety. For more severe cases of depression or anxiety (major depression, panic disorder, obsessive compulsive disorder and other more severe forms), I believe the advantage still lies with drugs. I am not dogmatic or fundamentalist either way - I believe in horses for courses.

You need to use the right tool for the job, and this is where supplements such as hypericum are under-utilised by those suffering mild to moderate cases. When using pharmaceutical drugs, there is a price to pay in terms of side-effects, so, considering that for mild to moderate cases hypericum matches drugs but with much milder side-effects (if any), in this scenario I believe the herbal treatment has a significant advantage.

It is important to note that a large number of people who start drug therapy soon quit due to intolerable side-effects. In many cases, these side-effects eventually settle down and fade, however for many people it is too hard to bear and they quit. Natural therapies such as hypericum have a much gentler start-up period, which means that, although it can take a little longer to have noticeable effects, people are unlikely to quit due to side-effects. I should also point out that this longer start-up period is another reason why natural options are not appropriate for more severe cases. If someone is severely depressed or even suicidal, their physici an needs to choose the therapy that will pull them out of their deep dark hole the quickest. Unfortunately, I would never, ever recommend natural therapies in such acute cases. If this describes you, please put down this eBook and seek immediate, professional attention. There are powerful, effective treatments that can quickly treat your current condition.

How does hypericum work?

Almost any antidepressant (whether drug or herb) works to relieve depression via the same basic mechanisms. Either -

1. Inhibiting the re-uptake of serotonin - This is how SSRI drugs (such as Prozac or Zoloft) work. These substances block the action of the serotonin transporter (SERT) which recycles serotonin back into the pre-synaptic neuron. By blocking the action of SERT, there is more serotonin floating around in the synapse between two neurons.

   Or

2. Inhibiting the action of monoamine oxidase - This is how monoamine oxidase inhibitors (MAOIs) work. Usually, monoamine oxidase breaks down serotonin, norepinephrine and dopamine so, by inhibiting its action, there are increased levels of all three monoamines in the brain.

Unfortunately there is no consensus as to exactly how hypericum exerts its beneficial effects on depression. Some researchers have claimed that it works as an SSRI, while others have indicated that it works as a MAOI. An in-vitro (i.e. - in a laboratory test-tube, not in an animal or human) study in 1994 found that hypericum clearly inhibited the action of monoamine oxidase when used at high doses. Similarly, studies conducted in 1997 and 1998 using even higher doses found that hypericum works at least partially as a MAOI. The problem with these high- dose studies is that they found no inhibition of monoamine oxidase using clinically relevant doses (ie - doses which roughly approximate what a person would typically take). So, while we know that hypericum functions as MAOI to at least some extent, it is unclear from these studies whether it functions as a MAOI at the dosages people are likely to take.

Likewise, several German studies in the 1990s found that hypericum inhibits the re-uptake of serotonin, norepinephrine and dopamine in-vitro, in a similar fashion to pharmaceutical antidepressants.

Animal studies have also all found a variety of effects, with no clear indication of a single mechanism underlying how exactly hypericum works. However the key point to draw from these and other studies is that hypericum consistently increases levels of serotonin, norepinephrine and dopamine in the brain. It's just that the relative degree to which each of these monoamines is increased or the proposed mechanism differs between studies.

Another interesting piece of the puzzle comes from sleep studies, which appear to indicate that hypericum has a similar impact on sleep architecture that pharmaceutical drugs have. Hypericum has been found to clearly suppress REM sleep in a similar fashion to SSRIs. The reason why this is so interesting is that there are many scientists who believe that there is a strong link between excess REM sleep and depression. When depressed patients participate in sleep studies, they are consistently found to have significantly more REM sleep (as a proportion of total sleep) than the rest of the population. What we do not yet know is - which is the chicken and which is the egg? Does depression causes excessive REM sleep or does excessive REM sleep cause depression? What we do know however, is that the normalising of REM sleep after commencing antidepressant therapy is strongly associated with an improvement in mood. So, could REM sleep suppression be one of the ways which hypericum works?

In-vitro and animal studies are one thing, however what about the subjective effects? Anecdotally, many users seem to feel that hypericum has a stronger effect on serotonin than the other monoamines. Particularly when compared to the two other most effective natural antidepressants - curcumin and rhodiola rosea, which appear to have a more broad-spectrum activity on all three.

That's the good news - what about the bad news?

While hypericum is generally an effective and potent natural antidepressant, it has one major downside - it affects how your body metabolises a variety of drugs. In fact, hypericum appears to affect almost any drug that is metabolised in the liver. Of particular concern is the impact on the blood-thinning drug warfarin.

Depending on the drug, hypericum can either increase or decrease the effectiveness of the particular medication. Therefore, if you are on any drugs at all, you need to clear things with your doctor before taking hypericum. In general however, I usually recommend that, if someone is taking any other medication, to first investigate curcumin and/or rhodiola rosea, as these don't have the same effects on other drugs

The only other potential side effect of note is increased photosensitivity. In a practical sense, this means that some people can become sunburned much more quickly than otherwise would have been the case if they were not taking hypericum. So I think it would be warranted to take a little extra precaution regarding sun exposure if you are taking hypericum.

The only other precaution (which applies to all herbal antidepressants) is to never combine hypericum with pharmaceutical antidepressants or any other drug that increases levels of serotonin, norepinephrine or dopamine. This can, in rare cases, lead to a life-threatening condition called serotonin syndrome. If in doubt, discuss with your primary care physician.

Dosage and recommended brands

The generally recommended dosage for hypericum is 300mg, 3 times a day, however with any psychotropic herb or pharmaceutical, I usually recommend people to start on a lower dose and work up. Hypericum is generally free of start- up problems, however it is always better to give your brain time to adjust. What I usually tell people is that you should never force your brain's neurochemistry. A little bit of something is good, but more is only better to a point. For example, if you are feeling depressed and you feel a bit better after a couple of weeks on the standard dose of hypericum, don't ever think that taking 10 times the dose will make you feel even better. It won't. The brain needs to be gently guided in the right direction, as if by a small rudder in your head. Suddenly push too hard in a different direction and you risk breaking the rudder. For example, by inducing serotonin syndrome (Don't worry, hypericum on its own has not been implicated in serotonin syndrome - this is just an example). Maybe start on 300mg, once in the morning and once in the afternoon, and then work up from there.

In terms of brands, I rarely ever recommend specific brands however in the case of hypericum, there are two stand-out brands available - Kira and Nature's Way Perika. However among these two, it tends to be completely unpredictable as to which you will find more helpful. I have often recommended people to try a month or two on one and then a similar time on the other to compare. The main difference is that some people find one of these two to be quite "relaxing" and the other "activating". There is no way to tell which one you will be so you may have to experiment.

Rhodiola Rosea

Rhodiola is a supplement I have been passionate about for a long time now, due to its unique mechanism of action and wide-ranging effects. Along with curcumin, rhodiola is one of my picks for supplements which will become increasingly well- known over the next ten years or so.

So what exactly is rhodiola rosea?

Rhodiola rosea is an herbal supplement which has been used for decades in Russian-block countries to treat what they refer to as 'nervous disorders', which encapsulates a range of conditions including stress, anxiety and depression.

However it has only recently risen to prominence in the West. In fact, there is even documented use all the way back to just after Christ lived! It is often referred to as an adaptogen, meaning it helps the body to recover from physical and mental stress.

Rhodiola rosea (also known as golden root or arctic root, among other things) is a plant that grows in cold areas of the northern hemisphere.

Rhodiola is most commonly associated with countries such as Russian and the other countries of the former USSR and has been reputedly used extensively by the Russian military to promote endurance.

In terms of prominence in the west, rhodiola rosea still lags far behind St.John's Wort, which enjoys far more popularity and widespread use. This is a pity, because rhodiola has a few advantages over St.John's Wort (which I will get to in a moment).

What is it used for and what is it believed to do?

- Note - Here I am talking about what conditions it is used to treat - not which conditions it is proven to treat. Sometimes there can be a huge difference between the two in both herbal medicine and traditional pharmaceutical medicine.
- Enhance the immune system
- Treat depression
- Improve endurance for physical activities
- Assist in weight-loss
- Improve sexual function
- Improve general energy levels
- Treat the effects of chronic stress

Now, let's look at these in more detail -

Rhodiola rosea belongs to a class of herbs known as adaptogens. Adaptogens are substances which restore homeostasis in the body. So if, for example, you are too wired and anxious, an adaptogen will calm you down. If you are lethargic and lacking energy, an adaptogen will give you energy.

Quite often, I am rather suspicious of adaptogens and the theory that underpins this class of supplements. There are quite a few natural therapies marketed as adaptogens which have very poor research-based evidence backing their use.

However rhodiola is one herbal medicine where there is not only a large body of anecdotal reports verifying the adaptogenic effects, but a good theoretical potential mechanism that would explain the effects.

By increasing levels of serotonin, norepinephrine and dopamine, rhodiola functions in a very similar way to a pharmaceutical antidepressant. If you are anxious depressed (high stress, high anxiety, poor sleep) and you take an antidepressant (such as an SSRI, tricyclic or MAOI) you will usually slowly begin to calm down and relax over time. If you are suffering from a more lethargic depression (low energy, hypersomnia, lack of motivation) and you take the same antidepressant, you will gradually start to spark up and feel more energetic. It is for this reason that, when people talk of the adaptogenic properties of rhodiola, what I believe they are really referring to is its ability to act as an antidepressant by increasing levels of the three primary monoamines.

Chronic stress is associated with a variety of tell-tale biomarkers, however the most emblematic marker of the condition is elevated cortisol levels. Cortisol is a vital hormone secreted by the adrenal cortex in times of stress. Cortisol is neither inherently good nor bad - it is just there to do a job. The problem is when you experience chronic stress associated with chronically elevated cortisol levels.

Cortisol is actually neurotoxic, however typically it is only secreted in small amounts for specific tasks such as dealing with stress and modulating your circadian rhythm (cortisol rises in the early morning to prepare you to wake up and drops in the evening to allow you to sleep). However if cortisol is allowed to run rampant, it can literally damage your brain - particularly the hippocampus. It just so happens that the hippocampus is the part of the brain that appears to suffer the most from depression and chronic stress. The hippocampi of depressed people can even have decreased mass compared to the general population! Fortunately,   the hippocampus is also amazingly plastic, so after successful recovery (possibly thanks to rhodiola), it usually returns to normal size and function.

The potent ability of rhodiola to decrease levels of stress hormones such as cortisol also leads to an unexpected additional benefit in the area of cardiac health.

Chronic stress is a known factor in a large proportion of all heart disease cases.

Chronically elevated levels of hormones and neurotransmitters such as cortisol and norepinephrine puts enormous stress on the heart. Reducing levels of norepinephrine and epinephrine in particular is vital for treating the greatest single risk factor for heart disease - high blood pressure. Whether by using beta-blockers such as propranolol (Inderal) or alpha-adrenal antagonists such as clonidine or guanfacine, the way to decrease blood pressure most effectively is by reducing levels of epinephrine and norepinephrine.

It is here where things get slightly complicated because, as you may have just thought - Isn't rhodiola supposed to increase levels of norepinephrine, not decrease? This is one of the seeming paradoxes of psycho-pharmacology - why do drugs that increase epinephrine eventually lead to reduced anxiety levels in some cases? For example, tricyclic antidepressants like amitriptyline increase levels of not only serotonin, but also norepinephrine. Patients on amitriptyline eventually report a dramatic decrease in anxiety. It is beyond the scope of this guide to go into too much detail however the key points are a) The sub-receptors of the adrenoreceptors (different sub-types have different functions) and b) the context - whether epinephrine is secreted as a stress response or a motivational response.

All this aside, the key point is that rhodiola appears to lower blood pressure and treat heart arrhythmias, leading to improved heart health. A study by Maslova et al found "Rhodiola rosea was ascertained to prevent both stress-induced catecholamine release and higher cAMP levels in the myocardium. Moreover, the adaptogen prevented lower adrenal catecholamines during stress. The findings suggest that the antistressor and cardioprotective effects of Rhodiola rosea are associated with limited adrenergic effect on the heart." The fact that rhodiola appears to limit the impact of stress on both the brain and heart is extremely interesting and something not replicated by too many pharmaceuticals or supplements.

Due to the fact that rhodiola increases levels of all three monoamines (serotonin, norepinephrine and dopamine), it tends to be a little more "activating" than the other popular antidepressant, St.John's Wort. Not surprisingly, I have therefore found it more helpful in cases of lethargic depression, rather than anxious depression. Norepinephrine (which is known as noradrenaline in some parts of the world) and dopamine are the two excitatory monoamines implicated in depression. Restoring levels of these two neurotransmitters will usually lead to improved energy levels, improved motivation and improved sexual function.

These just so happen to be some of the benefits attributed to rhodiola. You can see why the effects of rhodiola have not just been borne out in animal testing, but also make logical sense.

It is in the area of physical endurance that things get even more interesting. In various trials, rhodiola has been shown to improve recovery time (i.e. - shorten the time needed for recovery between two activities) and increase muscle strength. It appears to do this at least partially by increasing glycogen and protein synthesis.

For example, in a particular trial where students were broken into two groups (one group receiving rhodiola and one group receiving a placebo), the rhodiola group reported reduction in mental fatigue, better sleep quality, less requirement for sleep, more stable moods and increased motivation, far exceeding the placebo group.

So how exactly does rhodiola work?

Current research indicates that rhodiola functions primarily as a monoamine oxidase inhibitor (MAOI). Before SSRIs (such as Prozac and Zoloft), apart from tricyclic drugs, the only other option for treating depression was MAOIs. While MAOIs were extremely effective (they are considerably more effective than any modern-day antidepressant), they had a range of drawbacks. The most significant of these was the fact that while taking a MAOI, if you consumed food high in a substance called tyramine, you were at risk of a hypertensive crisis which could potentially be fatal. This, as you would expect, is a deal-breaker these days now that we have a range of safer options.

The beauty of several antidepressant supplements such as rhodiola and curcumin, is that they function as MAOIs but without the dangerous dietary risks. This is important to note, because without the danger component, MAOIs are excellent for treating depression due to their broad range of action. An SSRI like Prozac predominantly works to increase levels of serotonin only, while a MAOI increases levels of all three major monoamines. As you probably know, any substance that ends in "-ase" is usually an enzyme. Monoamine oxidase is an enzyme that breaks down serotonin, dopamine and norepinephrine for recycling. By inhibiting this enzyme, there is a greater number of these monoamines remaining in the synapse (the space between two neurons).

Interestingly, there are a range of anti-cancer benefits which have been proposed from the results of various studies. However, in general I feel uncomfortable touting anything as treating cancer so I won't go into any details. The research information I have seen is not yet compelling and only preliminary so please don't place any of your hopes with rhodiola for cancer.

Similarly I have seen claims regarding rhodiola's immune-boosting effects. Anything that improves mood and reduces stress will also improve immunity, so this is not particularly surprising. I don't think rhodiola is giving any boost to your immune system by another, direct route. I think by decreasing levels of cortisol, your immune response improves as an indirect result. The research on rhodiola and the immune system is not yet strong enough to make specific recommendations.

Likewise, the trials on rhodiola's effects on physical endurance have also been inconclusive. You could argue that improved mood and motivation would lead to improved physical performance. I can vouch for this personally. I tend to lose almost 100% of my tennis matches when I go into the match in a bad mood. Mind you, I don't win that much more when I am happy either. Apparently rhodiola can't fix a bad backhand!

However the effects of rhodiola on the brain are another case altogether. The research and clinical trial results for mood disorders and stress-related conditions have been extremely encouraging.

Due to the comparative lack of drug interactions, I usually recommend rhodiola rosea as the first option for treating depression. As it is a slightly newer supplement in the west, there isn't as much research yet compared to St. John's Wort, however what research is available has been generally positive. In particular, multiple rodent trials have demonstrated a clear ability to reduce some of the mental and physical effects of stress.

Most of the clinical research on rhodiola has focused on its ability to improve energy levels. For example, in a trial by Darbinyan et al, the authors concluded *"A statistically significant improvement in these tests was observed in the treatment group (RRE) during the first two weeks period. No side-effects were reported for either treatment noted. These results suggest that RRE can reduce general fatigue under certain stressful conditions."* (RRE is a particular extract of rhodiola).

Similarly, a study by Shevtsov et al found *"...a pronounced antifatigue effect..."* in the group taking an extract of rhodiola.

Whenever I want to assess the potential benefits of an herb or natural therapy, I look for meta-analyses where all the results from different trials are pooled together to get a more statistically significant indication of whether something works or not. A 2011 study did just this, and found that rhodiola appears to have benefit for physical and mental performance, along with mental health disorders.

Apart from the fact that rhodiola works on all three monoamines compared to St. John's Wort which just affects serotonin, rhodiola has another advantage.

St.John's Wort is a highly effective herbal antidepressant (in some countries it is the first line of treatment for depression) with little doubt as to its effectiveness. However it has one major problem - it affects the metabolism of just about any other drug you are taking. Depending on how you metabolise certain drugs, St. John's Wort can lead to either dramatically higher blood levels or dramatically lower levels. For example, St. John's Wort can increase the effects of certain sedatives while decreasing the effect of blood thinners such as Warfarin.

Decreasing the effects of Warfarin can be extremely dangerous and conceivably lead to lethal blood clots.

Therefore, my general recommendation to people is always - if you need to regularly take any other drug at the same time, St. John's Wort should be avoided.

Dosing

In terms of dose, like most things, start low and work your way up if necessary. I usually recommend a daily dosage of between 300-600mg, spread across two or three doses. In general, rhodiola has few negative side-effects. One to look out for is a mild stimulant effect (remember - it boosts levels of stimulating neurotransmitters norepinephrine and dopamine), so if you find it stimulating you may need to take your dose(s) before lunch time to avoid problems sleeping.

If people find that, after a few weeks they haven't improved, or if they are experiencing increased anxiety, I usually suggest a switch to St. John's Wort to get a more specific effect on serotonin.

One thing I should point out also is that you should only ever combine multiple drugs that affect neurotransmitters under the strict supervision of your primary care provider. So, for example, you should never combine rhodiola with an SSRI or other pharmaceutical antidepressant without the permission of your doctor or similar care provider. Occasionally this can lead to the rare condition known as serotonin syndrome, which can be fatal in some instances. Just because something is "natural", it doesn't mean that there aren't potential hidden dangers with misuse.

Some of the reputable brands for rhodiola include - Now Foods, Jarrow, Life Extension, Nature's Way and Thorne. Unlike St. John's Wort, no particular brand of rhodiola has significant benefits over another. This kind of experiential data should slowly emerge, but until then, any of the above brands should be fine. You may want to try each of them once to see if one works better than the other.

Magnesium

Recently, I have noticed that slowly magnesium is becoming the next 'hot' supplement, which, on the face of things seems rather strange at first glance. After all, magnesium is supposedly ubiquitous in our diet, with actual deficiency previously believed to be quite rare. However, research studies and anecdotal reports are emerging which appear to cast magnesium in a new light. In fact, in terms of unit sales, my guide to magnesium is my single biggest selling release on Amazon!

Up until a few years ago, I had always thought that magnesium helped treat anxiety for one reason - muscles need magnesium to relax. They use calcium to contract and magnesium to relax, which is why magnesium deficiency is associated with muscle tightness and cramping.
Also, for many years we have known about the relaxing effects of Epsom salts baths (Epsom salts is magnesium sulfate). To be honest, for many years I believed that Epsom salts were just placebo - that people were just getting relaxed by having a hot bath. Then I read a study that appeared to demonstrate that a large amount of magnesium is absorbed through the skin when we take an Epsom salts bath. This is now known as transdermal magnesium therapy and can be extremely effective in certain situations where oral magnesium is not recommended. There is also a growing minority of health professionals who believe that transdermal therapy is a much more effective way to treat a magnesium deficiency than taking oral supplements.

Originally I thought that magnesium helped anxiety because it aided in physical relaxation. As anyone who suffers anxiety will know, there is a feedback loop that occurs between anxious thoughts and physical sensations of anxiety. By breaking that feedback loop with magnesium, anxiety can dissipate. However, recently research has emerged showing a strong correlation between magnesium levels and serotonin levels. Low magnesium is now clearly linked with low serotonin. Not only this, but a certain study also concluded that for certain patients, magnesium therapy was as effective as antidepressant medication! Please don't take this as a signal to go off medication and start magnesium therapy as it depends on the person and the nature of the particular case of depression or anxiety. Magnesium supplements would do little to ameliorate suicidal depression. Nevertheless, it does point to a potentially potent alternative to antidepressant or antianxiety medications in certain scenarios.

One of the reasons I wanted to write this guide is that, as part of my research into the brain and body, I keep unearthing new research and new theories regarding magnesium. Along with omega 3 fatty acids and vitamin D, magnesium has the widest range of effects on the body of any substance, as I will now show.

So how do you know if you are deficient in magnesium? Symptoms can include anxiety, restless leg syndrome (RLS), sleep disorders, abnormal heart rhythms, blood pressure abnormalities, muscle spasms, weakness and insomnia.

However, if we are looking at potential applications for magnesium therapy, we need to first clarify what we are talking about. Magnesium therapy can either be used for correcting a medically-diagnosed deficiency or for treating a specific disorder. This is a key point as there are occasions where magnesium therapy can be helpful despite the lack of an actual deficiency. We can draw parallels with lithium, which is used to treat bipolar disorder, where we are not actually correcting a lithium deficiency per se. More on this in a minute.

Of all the nutrients, supplements and herbs that I have studied, magnesium has by far the longest list of potential applications. Magnesium therapy has demonstrated the ability to treat or ameliorate conditions such as – hypertension (high blood pressure), arthritis, type 2 diabetes, insomnia, problems with energy levels (due to ATP abnormalities), cholesterol problems, bladder spasms, menstrual cramps, muscle spasms and twitches, fibromyalgia, palpitations, heart arrhythmias, anxiety and panic attacks, DHEA deficiency plus a range of other nervous system, cardiovascular and musculoskeletal system problems.

Magnesium and the body

Magnesium is one of the most ubiquitous minerals in your body, with large amounts found in your bones, teeth, muscles and vital organs such as your heart and kidneys. Magnesium is required for more than 300 different biochemical reactions in your body including glucose metabolism, glutathione production, DNA creation and regulation of cholesterol production.

Magnesium is one of your most important co-factors. A co-factor is a chemical that is required for a particular biochemical reaction. So magnesium is important not just in its own right, but as a vital co-factor regulating everything from potassium to vitamin D.

The explosion of interest in magnesium over the past several years is due largely to one alarming fact – large proportions of the western world appear to be chronically deficient in magnesium. This is partly due to the fact that we are eating less of the healthy foods that are rich in magnesium, such as nuts and leafy green vegetables. Big Macs and KFC buckets (perhaps unsurprisingly) contain very little magnesium.

Rough estimates indicate that in the past century, our daily magnesium intake has halved. Considering the range of biological functions that magnesium is required for, it is little surprise that this is going to have downstream adverse effects. In terms of diet, it's not just the consumption of magnesium-poor foods that is the problem, but also the increasing consumption of foods made from grains. Grains contain substances called phytates (or phytic acid), which inhibit the process of absorbing magnesium. So while you may seem some outdated recommendations to increase your consumption of "magnesium-rich grains", this is misleading because you are not able to absorb much of the magnesium those grains contain. On the flipside, if you consume magnesium-rich leafy green vegetables like broccoli, you are getting magnesium delivered in a form you can absorb properly. This decrease in magnesium consumption is not just due to the types of food we are eating but also the magnesium that food contains. This means that even the amount of magnesium these supposed "rich" sources (such as grains) contain is decreasing due to the switch to magnesium-deficient fertilizers such as super- phosphate.

The other factor that I believe plays a part in widespread magnesium deficiency is chronic stress. During times of stress, your body liberates magnesium stores to be used for various emergency biological processes that are required for you to fight or flee (flight). If these stores of magnesium floating around your system are not required they are then excreted in your urine and lost. Chronic stress therefore unsurprisingly leads to magnesium deficiency. If we were to track the last century's decrease in magnesium consumption on a graph, I think we would also find a strong correlation with increased levels of chronic stress. A century ago, stress was strongly associated with the poor and downtrodden, whereas nowadays that correlation has broken down, with high-paid CEOs just as likely to be afflicted by chronic stress.

Not only is this chronic magnesium deficiency caused by decreasing amounts of magnesium in our diets, but also as a knock-on effect of the other major deficiency afflicting the western world – vitamin D. As I have mentioned in my other books, we are in the midst of a vitamin D deficiency epidemic that is implicated in everything from depression to inflammatorily-mediated heart disease. Your body needs adequate vitamin D to be able to absorb magnesium properly. This is no surprise when we look at the fact that plants also require magnesium to create energy from the sun via chlorophyll. Vitamin D and magnesium are closely linked.

Also closely linked to this is the role magnesium plays in your body's synthesis of steroid hormones – remember, vitamin D is not actually a vitamin, but more closely related to steroid hormones. As I mentioned in in my anti-aging book The Methuselah Project – How to live to 100 and beyond, DHEA is a steroid hormone often referred to as the "youth hormone" as levels decrease as you age. DHEA is so important in the fight against premature or accelerated aging that people are experimenting with artificially boosting DHEA via supplements (something I don't recommend by the way). The good news is that magnesium supplementation appears to boost DHEA levels, as magnesium is required for the synthesis of DHEA from cholesterol.

And while we are on the topic of cholesterol, magnesium appears to play a potentially beneficial role here as well, by functioning as a kind of natural statin. The synthesis of cholesterol in your body requires an enzyme known as HMG-CoA reductase. Statins, which are also known as HMG-CoA reductase inhibitors, work by inhibiting this process. So in cases where there is heightened risk of heart disease or medically-diagnosed hypercholesterolemia (pathologically high levels of LDL cholesterol), magnesium may provide similar protection as statins but without the side-effects. However, in the interests of disclosure I should point out that I believe statins should only be used in cases where there has already been a heart attack or where there is genuine hypercholesterolemia. Due to clever marketing, statins are now getting prescribed to those with mildly elevated cholesterol, where there is no demonstrated ability to protect against a heart attack. So, while magnesium shows the ability to inhibit HMG CoA reductase, I am yet to be convinced whether this is either beneficial or necessary.

However, another area where I genuinely do believe magnesium has a role to play in fighting disease is in the area of insulin resistance. As I mention regularly in my books, I believe one of the main causes of obesity, heart disease and certain other conditions is insulemic problems caused by consumption of quick-digesting carbohydrates such as bread and pasta. Magnesium is critically involved in the process of secreting insulin to deal with blood glucose. Magnesium deficiency has been associated with insulin resistance, poor glucose tolerance and impaired insulin secretion. The problem is that this creates a vicious cycle because insulin resistance is then associated with decreased levels of magnesium. This then leads to increased triglyceride levels (the part of a typical cholesterol test that is driven by the level of alcohol and dietary carbohydrate consumption), leading to increased risk of heart disease. My own opinion is that high triglyceride levels are a better predictor of heart disease than LDL numbers. Supplemental magnesium gives us a way to short-circuit this process.

Again on the subject of your cardiovascular system, another key point is that magnesium inhibits the constriction of your blood vessels, a major factor in the development of high blood pressure and incidence of stroke or heart attack. The cardiovascular system is where all physicians and researchers agree on the important of magnesium.

An important study from almost thirty years ago showed that the diuretics prescribed to treat hypertension were possibly leading to increased risk of heart problems due to the fact that they leeched magnesium and potassium. This means that these days, if you are on diuretic therapy with drugs such as hydrochlorothiazide, your doctor will usually also prescribe magnesium and potassium supplements.

To give you another sense of how important magnesium is for your heart, in certain cases where a patient is brought into the ER with a suspected heart attack, one of the first things that will happen is they will be given a large dose of magnesium intravenously to correct heart arrhythmias.

The benefits of magnesium for the heart are not just limited to emergency situations either. A ten year study found that eating a diet low in magnesium was associated with a 50 percent increase in risk of dying from a heart attack.

There is also a growing understanding of the role that magnesium plays in inflammatory conditions. Magnesium plays a vital role in controlling the cellular processes that lead to inflammation. As inflammation is gradually being identified as a causative factor in a range of disorders from depression to heart disease, by controlling inflammation with sufficient magnesium consumption, you are addressing the cause of a huge number of diseases and disorders. In The Methuselah Project, I recommended people get their c-reactive protein levels checked. C-reactive protein is your main biomarker for inflammation and is therefore commonly tested where there is an elevated risk for heart disease. A study by the Medical University of Carolina showed that there was a strong correlation between low levels of magnesium consumption and dangerously high levels of c-reactive protein.

As you may have heard, one of the reasons why magnesium increases levels of relaxation is that magnesium relaxes muscles at the cellular level. As I mentioned in the introduction, calcium drives the contraction (tensing) of muscles and magnesium plays the equal and opposite role. The problem is not, however, too much calcium per se, but too much calcium in proportion to magnesium. This leads to tense muscles, twitches and spasms.

However there is a more insidious problem with a high calcium to magnesium ratio. Magnesium plays a central role in allowing your body to properly absorb calcium. But magnesium doesn't work alone, and that's where vitamin D and vitamin K come in. There is a growing body of evidence that suggests that if you want to correct a vitamin D deficiency by taking large doses of vitamin D, you also need to take vitamin K supplements. The reason for this is that vitamin D (along with magnesium) is needed for the proper absorption of calcium. However, it is vitamin K that is needed to then allow your bones to absorb the calcium. In the absence of vitamin K or magnesium, that calcium can turn up in the worst possible place – your arteries. Calcium makes up a large proportion of the kind of arterial plaque that causes the problem we know as atherosclerosis. This is yet another reason to get your magnesium from vitamin K-rich leafy green vegetables instead of phytate-rich grains.

Those who have read my other books will know that I am leery of promoting anything as either a cure for or preventative of, cancer. The internet is already sufficiently clogged with morally bankrupt claims from people selling various unproven cancer treatments. Trust me, if any of those things worked, you would have read about it on the news. So while I would never claim that magnesium conclusively prevents cancer, there appears to be a definite association between low levels of magnesium consumption and rates of certain cancers. Studies in the US and Sweden appear to show that the higher the level of magnesium consumption, the lower the level of colon cancer incidence. It is far too early to draw any conclusions from these studies, however in the future this could be backed up by additional research that could give us a possible link between magnesium deficiency and cancer.

Premature aging caused by oxidative stress is so important that I dedicated a large proportion of The Methuselah Project to it. To bring you up to speed, oxidative stress is caused by free radicals which have an unpaired electron, causing damage at the cellular level as they try to steal electrons from other molecules.

Antioxidants fight this process by donating an electron without then becoming a free-radical themselves. Magnesium not only fights oxidative stress by protecting cells from heavy metals (such as mercury and lead, not Motley Crue or Whitesnake by the way) but also increases the ability of other antioxidants such as vitamin E and vitamin C to fight oxidative stress themselves. This is further highlighted by the fact that magnesium deficiency increases the production of free radicals and decreases production of the single greatest weapon against oxidative stress – glutathione.

Another scourge of modern times – PMS (pre-menstrual syndrome) has also been shown to have a strong correlation with not only low levels of magnesium, but low levels of magnesium in proportion to calcium. This may be due to the ability of magnesium to increase serotonin, or it could be the ability of magnesium to treat cramping due to its ability to relax muscles. Therefore it is no surprise that supplementing magnesium along with vitamin B6 has been shown to improve the symptoms of PMS.

A few studies have also shown that intravenous (not oral however) magnesium can be helpful in treating acute asthma attacks in children. It therefore comes as no surprise to note that a large study of more than 2000 children found a strong association between low levels of magnesium and asthma symptoms.

Another much smaller study found that a proprietary formulation containing magnesium reduced some of the pain commonly associated with this condition.

Recently magnesium has become a common treatment for migraine and tension- type headaches. Particularly in the case of tension headaches, this should come as no surprise. Drugs (such as anticholinergic muscle relaxants) used to treat tension headache do so by causing tense muscles in the head and neck to relax, creating exactly the same effect as magnesium achieves. Magnesium is cited as a possible treatment for and preventative of headaches as studies have shown a correlation between low levels of magnesium and certain types of headaches.

This should almost go without saying considering what we know about magnesium and your bones, however I should also point out that maintaining appropriate levels of magnesium is one of the most important factors (alongside vitamin D and vitamin K levels) for preventing osteoporosis and osteoarthritis.

Another common medical use of magnesium is in treating preeclampsia and eclampsia in pregnant women. This condition, which causes a dangerous spike in blood pressure during the third trimester, is usually treated with intravenous magnesium administered in the hospital.

Finally, another one of the most powerful uses of magnesium is for treating the extremely uncomfortable condition restless legs syndrome (RLS). Those who have never experienced RLS find it difficult to imagine why an uncomfortable sensation in your legs should be so debilitating. However RLS is not only exceedingly uncomfortable, it tends to strike when sufferers are trying to sleep, leading to secondary sleep problems. A small study (backed up by a large body of individual anecdotal reports) found that magnesium gives some relief from the symptoms of RLS. Interestingly, RLS is also a symptom of stopping opiate-based painkillers and this is where many of the anecdotal reports have come from. However I am not sure if RLS triggered by opiate withdrawal is underpinned by the same mechanism as the RLS usually experienced by the elderly.

Magnesium and the brain

New research is showing that magnesium is involved in a range of vital functions in the brain at the cellular level.

Magnesium functions as weak NMDA receptor antagonist, similar to the anti- dementia drug memantine and the OTC cough remedy dextromethorphan. The reason why memantine is an effective treatment (not a cure though, I should add) for dementia-type conditions such as Alzheimer's disease, points to one of the reasons why magnesium can be neuro-protective. NMDA receptor antagonists reduce excitatotoxicity caused by excessive glutamate and calcium activity. Think of excitatotoxicity like a jack-hammer, continuously activating a neuron without rest. If this process is not controlled, it leads to cell death. Expand this so it becomes a widespread phenomenon and dementia-related disorders can eventuate.

Magnesium (acting as an NMDA receptor antagonist) acts like a kind of nightclub bouncer, sitting on the neuron and guarding against glutamate and calcium- mediated activation. I should point out that glutamate and calcium are not inherently toxic, only becoming so when there is excessive activation leading to excitatotoxicity.

This ability of magnesium to prevent excitatotoxicity is not just limited to gradual long term problems either. Magnesium is believed to reduce the brain damage sustained during a stroke by reducing the massive amount of excitatotoxicity that is associated with this event. Not only does magnesium help in this context, high magnesium consumption is believed to confer a degree of protection against stroke in those people with hypertension.

As I mentioned in extensive detail in The Methuselah Project, the stress hormone cortisol is toxic for the brain and in particular, the hippocampus. This is believed to be the main reason why depressed subjects often have smaller hippocampi than non-depressed subjects. Fortunately, the hippocampus is arguable the most plastic part of your brain and can bounce back to normal with appropriate treatment.

It is magnesium's ability to attenuate the stress response (and the resultant neurotoxicity) that make it such a powerful anti-stress agent. Magnesium not only reduces the secretion of stress hormones such as ACTH (the hormone that drives cortisol release), but also reduces the extent to which these stress hormones can create downstream effects in the brain. Put another way, magnesium acts by putting the brakes on your stress response.

As magnesium is a cheap, widely available mineral that cannot be patented, we unfortunately don't have a large number of clinical studies regarding its use in mood disorders or brain function. The trials that have been conducted however, have shown benefit in treating premenstrual dysphoric disorder, chronic fatigue and mania.

Dosage and available forms

Magnesium is a little more complicated than most other supplements due to the fact that it not only comes in a range of forms, but also can be either administered orally (with a tablet or capsule) or transdermally (absorbed through the skin).

There is a bit of controversy in magnesium circles (assuming there is such a thing as a "magnesium circle" of people) regarding oral versus transdermal. On one side you have some physicians who feel that not enough magnesium gets absorbed transdermally and on the other side you have those who believe that transdermal absorption is more effective as it bypasses the digestive process.

The first thing I will say (and on this point everyone agrees) is that you should try to get as much magnesium as possible from whole foods such as leafy green vegetables and nuts. With whole foods you often find that magnesium is bound with a range of synergistic vitamins and minerals such as vitamin K. However, while magnesium consumption in whole foods will help prevent a diagnosable deficiency, it may not be enough to actually treat or prevent a specific illness.

In terms of all the different forms of magnesium available, my opinion is that you are 95% better than you would have been just by taking any magnesium supplement. Then, arguably, you may get some additional benefits by taking a particular type of magnesium. The main available forms are –

Magnesium glycinate – A chelated form generally believed to be the most bioavailable.

Magnesium oxide – A non-chelated form that is the most commonly used in supplements due to low cost

Magnesium citrate – A form with citric acid that is also used as a laxative

Magnesium threonate – A more recent development which is showing initial promise due to its superior ability to get inside you mitochondria (your cellular powerhouse). There is also some emerging research indicating that this form has a particular ability to improve cognitive function, however it is too early to tell conclusively.

Magnesium sulfate – Commonly known as Epsom salts and is an excellent source for transdermal absorption.

Magnesium chloride – The form used in magnesium oil and in intravenous preparations.

In terms of dosage, you can start around 200-400mg (depending on the form – the dose will be adjusted by the manufacturer depending on the form used) per day and then work up from there with doctor's orders. I usually recommend getting your doctor's OK before starting any new supplementation program because your ability to tolerate supplements will depend on your other medications and your physical health. For example, medium to large dose daily magnesium therapy is not recommended for the infirm or for anyone with kidney problems. Your kidneys process any excess magnesium, preventing issues with toxicity – hence they need to be functioning properly to tolerate large doses of magnesium.

A good gauge as to how much is too much is whether you start to experience diarrhea. Too much magnesium will cause a laxative effect, so you may need to reduce the oral dosage and try transdermal magnesium therapy.

One of the main problems we have in identifying magnesium deficiency is the difficulty we have in accurately measuring levels. The amount circulating in your blood stream is only a small proportion of overall levels. For example, most of your magnesium is stored away in your bones. In this way magnesium is similar to serotonin, another substance where we don't have any reliable way to measure levels as a diagnostic tool. This is why often, magnesium deficiency (like serotonin deficiency – assuming this exists) is diagnosed via symptoms rather than a blood test.

In terms of transdermal absorption, your options are either Epsom salts baths or rubbing magnesium oil (as magnesium chloride) on to the skin.

As magnesium relaxes the muscles and increases serotonin, it also has a great reputation as a sleep enhancer. Therefore it makes sense to take it before bed.

There are a range of different ways you can take it, so perhaps aim for a nice balanced mix. You can either take Epsom salts baths, magnesium supplements or eat a diet high in magnesium. Foods high in magnesium include - tofu, legumes, whole grains, green leafy vegetables, Brazil nuts, soybean flour, almonds, cashews, pumpkin and squash seeds, pine nuts, and black walnuts.

Here is an ideal magnesium boosting activity – Enjoy a meal with plenty of leafy greens and some nuts before heading down to the beach for a long soak in the ocean. First you get the dietary magnesium bound with synergistic vitamin K, then you get to absorb magnesium transdermally from the seawater while boosting levels of vitamin D from the sun exposure. Just remember to keep your direct (sunblock free) skin exposure to around 20 minutes or less to avoid burning and increasing your risk of skin cancer.

SAM-e

SAM-e is another popular antidepressant alternative which may be worth investigating. As I just mentioned, depression can be caused by all kinds of different things. SAM-e addresses one part of your brain's activity and if this part (called methyl group transfers for those interested in looking into it in more detail) is dysfunctional, you may get some benefit. The exact mechanism of action is unclear however it is believed that for some people, a shortage of SAM-e in the brain can cause problems with the synthesis of serotonin. A bonus of SAM-e is that it has also been shown to improve symptoms of arthritis, while the major downside is that it can be expensive. A cheaper alternative is to supplement with trimethylglycine ("TMG"), which is believed to have similar effects as SAM-e supplementation.

L-Methylfolate

L-Methylfolate is a form of the common vitamin supplement folate, which women are usually encouraged to take while pregnant to prevent neural tube defects in their baby. Unfortunately a certain subset of the population are unable to convert folate to l-methylfolate, which is a big problem as folate is a vital co-factor for your brain's production of serotonin. These people lack the gene for MTHFR, an enzyme needed to convert folate into the active form. This is such a powerful driver of serotonin levels, that several companies have patented forms of l-methylfolate as treatments for depression. The target market for the pharmaceutical version of l-methylfolate is the group of people who are taking SSRI medication but not seeing any improvement. Often, adding l-methylfolate (as a supplement or the pharmaceutical version) can make all the difference.

However you need to bear in mind that if you have no issues with your ability to produce l-methylfolate from folic acid, you will see little additional benefit from adding this supplement to your regime. However, if you think you may have an issue with this conversion process or be naturally low in dietary folate, I think it makes more sense to supplement with l-methylfolate than with folic acid if you are looking to optimise brain function.

Curcumin

It is testament to the amazing properties of curcumin that it is one of the few substances to feature both in the "Cognition" section of this guide and the "Mood" section. Also, due to the range of effects, it is the only one I have decided to mention twice – this time focusing on the mood-elevating aspects.

Curcumin is the rising superstar in the field of natural depression treatments. In fact, curcumin is the rising star in multiple fields now - not just depression. I am such a massive supporter of curcumin that I dedicated a whole guide to it.

Curcumin is extracted from turmeric, one of the key ingredients in an Indian curry. So, as you would expect, curcumin has a long history of use in traditional Indian and Chinese medicine.

Curcumin appears to be beneficial for anxiety and depression for two reasons.

Firstly, it functions as one of the most powerful natural anti-inflammatories available. In some tests it works almost as well as an anti-inflammatory painkiller such as ibuprofen. There is a growing school of thought that mental disorders are strongly associated with increased levels of inflammation in the brain and body. What isn't yet clear is which way the arrow of causation goes. Does inflammation cause mental problems or do mental problems cause inflammation? Irrespective of the answer, it appears that curcumin exerts at least some of its beneficial effects by reducing inflammation in the brain.

In animal studies, curcumin has also shown the ability to regrow cells in the hippocampus. Remember, depression is associate with a loss of mass in the hippocampus and effective depression treatments are usually associated with an increase in hippocampal mass.

Curcumin also demonstrates an ability that is extremely rare in the world of supplements - the ability to increase levels of BDNF. Again, BDNF is strongly associated with important repair work in the depressed or anxious brain.

However the main way that curcumin works is that it also functions as a MAOI (monoamine oxidase inhibitor), leading to increased levels of serotonin, dopamine and norepinephrine

Remember, this is not just "out there" left field theorizing. The benefits of curcumin are being recognised in various medical journals around the world. For your reference, I have put an extract of a study from the Indian Journal of Pharmaceutical Sciences here.

Vitamin B6

Like folate, B6 is another co-factor in the production of serotonin. Think of co- factors like things you add into a beaker for a science experiment. To make serotonin, you need the base (l-tryptophan) and various co-factors (such as folate and B6) before you will see a small puff of smoke coming out of the beaker to tell you that serotonin has been made. (Note - this is just an analogy - I am not talking about actually making serotonin in a beaker or there being a puff of smoke when serotonin is made!)

Instead of taking all the individual B-group vitamins, apart from l-methylfolate, I recommend you just take a single "Multi-B" that has all the B-group vitamins in it. Remember, mental stress like the type associated with anxiety and depression, depletes your stores of B-group vitamins, so I always recommend people take a single Multi-B if they are under any stress.

Tryptophan/5-htp

As I mentioned earlier, serotonin is made from the amino acid l-tryptophan. You may have heard of l-tryptophan in those stories that sometimes circulate as to why a big turkey meal (at Thanksgiving) makes you sleepy. In turns out that this is just a myth. While turkey does contain l-tryptophan, there is nowhere near enough to cause any noticeable change in mood or energy.

When serotonin is made, it goes through several steps. Firstly, l-tryptophan is converted into 5-htp. Then 5-htp is converted into serotonin.

Both l-tryptophan and 5-htp are available as supplements. In general, as 5-htp is one step closer to actual serotonin, it is believed to be a more potent method to increase levels of serotonin.

For both of these supplements, the results tend to be hit and miss. Some people swear by 5-htp while others get no benefit. The reason is that depression and anxiety are not one single illness with a single cause. 5-htp will be beneficial if you have an issue with having enough l-tryptophan in your diet. Alternatively, some people consume a high protein diet which is much higher in l-tyrosine than l- tryptophan. High levels of l-tyrosine tend to prevent l-tryptophan from crossing the blood brain barrier, leading to higher levels of dopamine and lower levels of serotonin. If low dopamine is your issue, this is great, however if low serotonin is the cause of your issues, this can be problematic.

Fortunately, 5-htp is relatively cheap and with few side-effects, so there is rarely little to lose by trying it out. I usually recommend starting on 100mg a day (50mg after lunch and 50mg before bed), before slowly moving up to 200mg a day. The optimum dosage for 5-htp is also unpredictable, so some experimentation may be required to get the dose correct.

Inositol

If 5-htp increases the building blocks of serotonin, inositol improves serotonin's ability to move between neurons. Inositol makes up the fatty component of your brain (along with omega 3 fatty acids and phosphatidylserine (among other things).

Most research into inositol has been focused on obsessive compulsive disorder (OCD), panic disorder and bi-polar disorder, however there has also been good anecdotal reports of benefit for other anxiety disorders as well.

Most "Multi-Bs" will also contain inositol, however in smaller doses. Another option is a combination supplement which contains choline and inositol. The reason why choline is often combined with inositol is that research has shown they have a synergistic effect (1+1=2+x). Also, a recent study showed a strong link between low levels of choline in the diet and levels of anxiety.

Depending on what is behind your current issues, inositol could be either extremely helpful or little help at all. However, consumption of inositol has only beneficial effects on the brain so there is little downside to giving it a try. Either just get by on the amount included in your Multi-B, or take a single "choline plus inositol" capsule per day.

Omega 3 Fatty Acids

Omega 3 supplements (in the form of fish oil or krill oil) have become the most popular supplements in the world for a good reason. Omega 3 supplements are almost unique in the fact that, if you aren't an Inuit or living on a diet based exclusively on seafood, you should be taking Omega 3 supplements each day.

What you probably didn't know, is that Omega 3 supplements have also been extensively studied for various mental disorders with positive results. However, despite the fact that you probably should be taking Omega 3, not everyone will get noticeable improvement in their mood disorder from taking them. The reason is that, as I mentioned previously, it depends on what is causing your anxiety or depression that dictates what will help you get better.

Like inositol, Omega 3 appears to improve cell membrane permeability, which enables your neurons to communicate more effectively with one another. If faulty or impaired neurotransmission is behind your problems, Omega 3 supplementation could be extremely effective.

Omega 3 is also vital for another reason - it is a potent anti-inflammatory. In your brain and body, to a certain degree, inflammation is controlled by Omega 6 (which increases inflammation) and Omega 3 (which decreases it). Remember, inflammation is not dangerous in itself - without inflammation your body would not be able to heal certain injuries and fight illness. The problems only emerge when the balance between Omega 3 and Omega 6 gets of out of whack. The theory as to why inflammation today runs rampant in humans is that in the past, our diets were more skewed to Omega 3. However today, with our grain-based diet, we consume far too much Omega 6 and not enough Omega 3. Not only do we consume a large amount of grain, our animals are now also mainly fed grains and oilseeds (corn, wheat, barley, soybean meal) instead of grass, so our meat is also now high in Omega 6.

There is a fascinating area of research recently which hypothesizes that depression may be associated with elevated levels of inflammation in the brain. As this is early days, scientists don't yet know whether inflammation causes depression or whether depression causes inflammation, however it is certainly a promising line of inquiry. Due to the fact that many sufferers of depression have indicated that Omega 3 appears to help them, this would make perfect sense.

This also appears to be the case for bipolar disorder (manic depression), which is associated with dramatic mood swings and shifts in perception of reality. Many doctors are now supplementing patients with Omega 3 along with their standard pharmaceutical treatments. I need to stress here that in no circumstances should someone read this and think that they can stop taking their mood-stabilizing medication and switch to fish oil. As you have no idea how you will react, this would be incredibly dangerous. If you are interested in the use of fish oil for bipolar disorder, discuss with your doctor.

My preference is to get your Omega 3 from a wide-range of sources. Omega 3 contains two important substances - DHA and EPA. Each source of Omega 3 has different ratios of these two substances and different levels of absorption by your body. The most common sources of Omega 3 include - Fish Oil, Krill Oil, Cod Liver Oil* (which also contains Vitamin D and Vitamin A), Seafood** (particularly fatty fish), Grass-Fed Beef and Eggs. As a bonus, krill oil contains a powerful antioxidant called astaxanthin which has on its own been shown to exert beneficial effects on the brain.

* Due to the fact that cod liver oil also contains Vitamin A, you should be careful to keep your consumption of this at reasonable levels. In some instances, high levels of Vitamin A can be toxic for humans. More is not always better.

** Be careful to keep your consumption of certain fish that are high in mercury to sensible levels. In general, fish at the top of the food chain such as sharks, tuna or swordfish, are the main offenders you need to be careful of.

Short-term fixes to help you relax

This section will focus on short term solutions to anxiety which enable you to calm down, relax and begin to heal. Whilst anxiety responds extremely well to drugs and supplements quite quickly, depression is entirely different. Apart from recreational drugs (which, I shouldn't have to tell you, should be entirely avoided if you have any mood disorder whatsoever) or prescription painkillers, there are not a lot of options for improving your mood through taking a pill. Improving your mood takes work (on your thoughts and behaviours) and time. This is beyond the scope of this book, however I recommend books like Brain Renovation or Mindfulness for Beginners if you are interested in the behavioral and cognitive aspect of healing your depression.

One quick note before I proceed – Originally I included Jamaican Dogwood in the below list, however I have decided to remove it because I am a little concerned with toxicity. Used in normal amounts, it is usually quite safe, however there is the ability to take too much, which can lead to trouble. If the safety information changes or new research emerges I will include it. There is already such a wide range of safe options that I don't think excluding it from this list narrows your options dramatically. Likewise, I can't include Kava, due to similar questions regarding long-terms safety.

Also, there are supplements here which appear promising but do not yet have enough research backing. For example, hops (yes, the same hops from beer!) appears to improve sleep quality, however there are no proper studies on hops to measure its effects or mechanism of action. There is a single study which showed that hops combined with valerian appeared to improve sleep quality compared to placebo. However, in this study hops was combined with valerian so it is difficult to tell where the effect came from. If new research emerges, I will include other supplements such as hops.

Similarly, there are herbs and supplements which possibly do work to increase relaxation but are not sufficiently potent enough to recommend. Herbs such as chamomile fit into this category. With chamomile, it is difficult to separate actual effects from placebo effects which may be experienced due to the act of slowly enjoying a nice up of tea.

Valerian

In terms of relaxant herbs, nothing comes close to valerian for popularity – and for good reason too. Any herbal "chill pill" or sleep aid will almost definitely have valerian as one of the components. If you are looking to improve sleep and relax, valerian should almost always be one of your first options.

As I have mentioned, most relaxants and sedatives work by increasing levels of GABA. Valerian appears to do this by inhibiting the breakdown of GABA, which leads to higher levels of the brain.

By far my favourite aspect of valerian is the fact that it works to dampen down the activity of your amygdala. The amygdala is central to your "fight or flight" response, by deciding what is possible dangerous (or important in other ways) and acting as your early warning system. Have you ever been walking through a forest or bushland and thought you saw a snake? You no doubt jumped back, heart racing, before moments later realising it was a stick on the ground. You can thank your amygdala for that. The amygdala is involved in almost all cases of anxiety and depression, so by dampening down any overactivity, you should see measurable improvements in your condition.

Most studies on valerian are focused on its effects as a sedative. In most of these studies, valerian improved all the aspects of sleep (time to fall asleep, times awakened, duration of sleep and sleep quality) compared to placebo.

My one concern regarding valerian is just how close it is to a benzodiazepine. Benzodiazepines are notoriously toxic for the brain in high doses or after long term use. In fact, any drug or supplement that modulates GABA should almost always be considered a short-term fix. Valerian fits into this category so I believe you should view it as a short term solution to insomnia or a week or so of stress relief. Just like any sleeping tablet, it is not healthy to become reliant on valerian to get a good night's sleep.

Passionflower

Along with valerian, passionflower is probably the most widely used herbal relaxant in the world today. The majority of supplements marketed as relaxants will have passionflower as one of the components.

As expected, passionflower exerts its effects mainly by increasing levels of GABA in the brain, just like benzodiazepine drugs. In fact, much of the clinical research regarding passionflower is focused on comparing it against pharmaceutical sedatives. In fact, a 2007 study found that passionflower reduced anxiety to a similar degree as midazolam (a benzodiazepine). Likewise, a study by the University of Florida found that passionflower reduced anxiety to the same degree as diazepam.

I have to make a point, however. After reading the research on passionflower I was quite amazed and a little sceptical. As someone who has taken both passionflower and benzodiazepines (as sleeping tablets), I have never felt the same degree of potency with the herbal option. Put another way, after taking passionflower, I feel definitely relaxed and calm, whereas benzodiazepines completely knock me out. Therefore I am more than curious to note how these research studies found the anti-anxiety effects to be similar.

While I doubt that the potency of passionflower matches a pharmaceutical sedative, it has an important clear advantage. The quality of your sleep on passionflower is dramatically better than with benzodiazepines. You wake up feeling refreshed and energetic.

Like all herbs, passionflower can also have a wide variation between brands, so some experimentation may be required to find a brand with acceptable potency. The safety profile of passionflower is excellent so don't be afraid to dose slightly more aggressively than the recommended dosage on the bottle.

Ashwagandha (Withania Somnifera)

Ashwagandha is an herb with a long history of use in traditional Indian Ayurvedic medicine which has some really interesting properties. I can't think of many supplements that can act as a relaxant, an antidepressant and a cognitive- enhancing nootropic.

The research backing for ashwagandha is impressive. One study showed that the anti-anxiety effect of ashwagandha was similar to the benzodiazepine lorazepam (Ativan) and another showed antidepressant effects similar to the tricyclic antidepressant imipramine.

Ashwagandha also functions as an anti-stress adaptogenic herb (similar to ginseng), which appears to neutralise some of the neuro-toxic aspects of chronic stress. In a fascinating 2001 clinical study, rats were exposed to chronic stress to mimic the type of physiological reactions seen when humans are stressed. The rats treated with ashwagandha had around 80% less neural degeneration than the rats which were not treated!

One of the worst aspects of chronic stress on the brain is via the stress hormone cortisol. Cortisol is a vital part of how your body deals with acute stress; however when stress become chronic, cortisol becomes toxic for the brain. In another interesting study, ashwagandha was shown to have dramatic and measurable effects on decreasing levels of cortisol. There are not many supplements which have this direct effect on cortisol, which makes ashwagandha one of the more interesting supplements available for treating chronic stress.

The other thing that makes ashwagandha a little unique is the fact that I could have easily included it in this section on relaxants/sedatives or I could have included it in Part 1, due to its ability to slowly heal the brain by reducing cortisol levels.

This ability of ashwagandha to physically repair the brain has also been validated in a clinical study that demonstrated measurable increases in the regeneration of brain cells. It is for this reason that ashwagandha is also being investigated as a novel treatment for Alzheimer's.

Lemon Balm (Melissa officinalis)

Lemon Balm, which is a member of the mint family, is another herb with a long history as a relaxation and stress-buster. In a study with human subjects, administration of lemon balm lead to not insignificant increases in self-reported levels of calmness.

As with most of the other herbs in this section, lemon balm also works by inhibiting the breakdown of GABA in the brain, leading to reduced anxiety, increased calmness and improved sleep quality.

However, where lemon balm appears to differ is via its ability to improve mood and cognitive ability by modulating acetylcholine receptors. Acetylcholine is central to cognitive ability and memory recall. Drugs used to treat Alzheimer's usually work by increasing the activity of acetylcholine. Promisingly, a small study showed that lemon balm provided modest benefit in patients with early-stage Alzheimer's.

In terms of sleep quality, the problem with the research on lemon balm is that it is usually studied in combination with other agents (such as valerian or passionflower). However, the majority of these studies found a definite advantage over placebo. Therefore, we cannot infer that lemon balm is proven to help with sleep and anxiety-related problems on its own, just in combination with other herbs, it does tend to work. Therefore, the no-brainer solution is to target combination products which combine lemon balm with a range of other herbs.

Skullcap

Another good modulator of GABA is skullcap. Along with valerian and passionflower, skullcap is the other herb mostly like to be included in any sedative or relaxation preparation.

Various compounds (mainly baicalin and baicalein) in skullcap appear to bind to the benzodiazepine GABA receptors, leading to increased levels of relaxation and improved sleep.

In terms of quality research, skullcap lags a little behind others such as valerian. It would be good to see some additional research on the mechanism of action and any differences between skullcap and other herbal options.

In the meantime, all we have to go on is a few studies (which have generally been positive for skullcap as a relaxant and sedative) and anecdotal reports supporting skullcap as an effective herb.

An important point

If I was to give one piece of advice for all the relaxation supplements mentioned in this section it would be – Use drugs on the rare occasion when you are desperate (suffering from insomnia before an important day, severe anxiety or a panic attack) and use supplements on a more regular basis to help you dim down low level anxiety, arousal or stress levels. During a full-blown panic attack, any of the supplements and herbs mentioned here are going to be of little use. So please don't read this guide and flush your important medication down the drain. Repair your brain slowly by increasing serotonin and then hopefully at some point in the future (with your doctor's OK), you will be able to ceremoniously and dramatically flush your drugs down the toilet. Patience is required.

Mood Food

All the supplements in the world are not going to help if you are also eating garbage. It's like starting a fire at the same time as you are trying to put one out. Putting high-quality fuel into your brain's "tank" is vital for first recovering and then thriving.

So, firstly, what do we already know based on current research (and what is mentioned in this guide)?

- You need a balanced source of protein to get the amino acids needed to produce serotonin (l-tryptophan) and dopamine/norepinephrine (l- tyrosine/l-phenylalanine)

- You need plenty of magnesium. The Standard American Diet ("SAD") is notoriously low in magnesium

- The SAD is well-known for having far too many simple carbohydrates in the form of - sugar, bread, pasta, French fries etc.

- The SAD is also typically low in Omega 3 fatty acids and at the same time, far too high in Omega 6 fatty acids. We don't eat enough seafood (Omega 3) and the meat we eat tends to be fed with grain and is therefore much higher in Omega 6 than our bodies evolved to tolerate.

- Depression is associated with increased levels of oxidative stress. Oxidative stress is basically damage that occurs in the brain and body as a result of natural processes and reactions. Normally your body has various ways of keeping this oxidative stress in relative check. However, when you put additional stress on your brain (depression) and don't consume a diet rich in antioxidants (which, as the name suggests, fight oxidation), oxidative stress can get out of control, rapidly aging your brain

So therefore, we need to follow some rough guidelines for ensuring that we put the right fuel in the tank to fight depression and anxiety. I have tried to make the following section as succinct and easy to follow as possible, so I have created a list of guidelines for you to keep in mind when constructing your new "diet". By "diet", I don't mean a crash course short term fix to lose weight, whereupon you then return to your old ways. I mean a sustainable, long term change in your eating habits to gradually return your brain to its natural, healthy state.

3. Where possible, less red meat, more seafood. Seafood is high in Omega 3 and low in Omega 6. Try to concentrate more on wild-caught seafood than farmed. Farmed fish is often fed entirely with Omega 6-rich commercial feed products. Minimise consumption of fish at the top of the food chain such as shark, tuna or swordfish, which can often be high in mercury (mercury concentrates with each step up the food chain). The best sources of seafood are sardines, salmon and oysters (oysters are the richest known source of zinc, another important mineral for your brain)

4. When eating red meat, where possible try to go for grass fed rather than grain fed. Grass fed meat is much higher in Omega 3.

5. As a general dietary rule, your diet should have the following structure -

- Unlimited vegetables - particularly leafy green vegetables like broccoli which are high in folate and other brain-healthy substances
- Plenty of high quality animal protein
- Plenty of high quality fats (more on this in a minute)
- Restrict whole grains (wheat, barley, oats)
- Plenty of fruit. However this doesn't mean unlimited fruit, as certain fruit can be high in fructose, which is not good for the brain.

6. Try to eliminate trans-fats completely from your diet as these have no benefits and only negative effects on the brain and cardiovascular system. Thankfully, trans-fats are slowly being reduced from foods nowadays. Depending on your country, trans-fats may have different names on the ingredients list of products such as cookies or deep fried items. For example, trans-fats can be called "partially hydrogenated vegetable oil" or similar.

7. Don't believe the old warnings regarding saturated fats. For most people, Omega 6 fatty acids are a much bigger problem. It still amazes me that many people think that margarine could be healthier than grass-fed butter. Your brain needs saturated fat for a variety of processes. For example, saturated fat is vital for vitamin D synthesis and transport into your brain

8. Likewise, reduce consumption of omega 6 rich vegetable oils (canola, soybean etc.) when cooking and switch towards either butter or olive oil. There is often debate about saturated fat versus polyunsaturated, however one thing that everyone agrees is that olive oil is extremely healthy.

9. Try to completely eliminate any flavoured drink from your diet. This includes sodas, fruit juices and alcoholic drinks. I understand that many people love their beloved alcohol, however not only is alcohol rapidly converted into sugar, but it plays havoc with your neurotransmitters. Also, one of the greatest health myths there is, is that fruit juice is healthy. A single orange is healthy, a glass of orange juice made from 5 oranges with all the fibre removed, is NOT healthy. Fruit juice is virtually pure sugar and is terrible for your brain and mood. You will get a quick spike in energy followed by a prolonged crash.

The Best Mood Foods in the World

The following is a list of the best, commonly available foods in the world. Note that I have focused on easily available foods. Naturally, there are a myriad of exotic and obscure foods that are extremely healthy but out of reach of most. I have therefore focused on foods commonly available to most of the Western world.

- Leafy green vegetables - broccoli, cabbage, asparagus (Essentially any leafy green is good for you though

- Eggs - Nature's superstar food. Packed with a range of brain healthy substances such as choline and vitamin D. Don't worry about cholesterol (which your brain needs anyway). Even if you do believe that high cholesterol causes heart disease, there is an extremely weak link between dietary cholesterol and serum cholesterol levels.

- Fruit - Berries are the superstars of the fruit world as they are packed with unique antioxidants for brain repair. Focus on - blueberries, raspberries, strawberries, blackberries. Also, cherries are great for reducing inflammation.

- Seafood - Any seafood is good for you however I believe sardines, salmon and oysters are particular superstars.

- Whole oats - Strict paleo types may disagree however I think whole oats eaten as porridge or oatmeal are much healthier than other grain-based alternatives such as puffed wheat, corn flakes or rice puffs. However try to restrict the amount of oats you eat. While they contain healthy goodies like beta-glucan, the protein in oats (avenin), is similar to gluten and not particularly good for you. However at the end of the day, I am not fundamentalist about this. Some people can tolerate avenin (or gluten), while others cannot. You will soon find out where you stand with oats.

- Grass fed meat – This not only gives you a great source of animal protein but also reduces your overall Omega 6 load, as the meat is not raised on grain

- Prunes - High in sugar (so only a small quantity should be eaten) but packed with a range of brain-healthy substances

- Natural/Greek Yoghurt - Packed full of healthy gut bacteria which help you to absorb certain brain-friendly vitamins from your diet.

- Red capsicum/peppers - Very high in Vitamin C

- Ginger - natural anti-inflammatory

- Avocado or olives for healthy fats

- Nuts – particularly walnuts, almonds and pecans. Excludes peanuts (which aren't actually nuts)

Exercise turns on a light in your brain

Exercise is the single greatest thing you can do for your brain. And evolution knows it too, which is why there is a complex system of biochemical reactions that reward you when you exercise.

You have probably heard of the runner's high right? You have probably also heard that jogging can make you high because of endorphins, your body's own internal morphine. Well, it turns out that this is only partly true. But I'll get to that in a bit.

In terms of building a super-brain, the single most important factor is relating to BDNF (brain-derived neurotrophic factor), your brain's own "miracle-gro" (as I have heard a few other authors refer to it as). I mentioned BDNF a few times earlier in this guide, but in order to explain the benefits of increased BDNF, I need to go into a little more detail.

BDNF is a protein that helps your existing brain cells to thrive and also helps drive important aspects of neurogenesis – the birth of new neurons. Neurogenesis seems so commonplace nowadays that it is easy to forget that up until only a few years ago it was believed that neurogenesis was impossible. Remember being told that you are born with a certain number of brain cells and can never grow new ones? Well, it turns out that was incorrect.

It also turns out that exercise is the single most powerful behaviour you can engage in to stimulate the secretion of BDNF in important parts of the brain such as the hippocampus. The hippocampus is central to a sharp brain (particularly memory recall) and a good mood. The hippocampus of depressed people is often found to have actually shrunk by a measurable amount! The good news is that, of all the areas in your brain, the hippocampus is one of the best at recovering and growing new neurons.

In terms of exercise for neural functioning, there is a great body of work centred on dementia patients, such as those with Alzheimer's. As I often mention, research on Alzheimer's gives us great indications regarding what works to improve cognition and memory.

Therefore, it is unsurprising that multiple studies have shown that exercise improves aspects of dementia both acutely and chronically. What this means is that a single episode of exercise (say, jogging for 30 minutes) increases production of BDNF and improves markers of cognition (acutely), while a continued exercise program gives additional benefits which gradually accumulate (chronically).

However it is in the area of depression and anxiety treatment that exercise has the most research behind it.

In his book Jump Start, Benjamin Kramer says *"Study after study has clearly shown that cardiovascular exercise and/or weight training works just as well as antidepressant medication, but with one key advantage - Those subjects who treat their anxiety and depression with exercise tend to stay well, whereas those who treat their depression with medication have a significantly higher relapse rate"*.

Likewise, in his book Spark, John Ratey cites compelling evidence which clearly demonstrates the link between exercise and not only mood, but cognitive function also. If you are serious about understanding the nexus between exercise and brain health, I strongly urge you to read books such as Ratey's. He was trying to get the message out about this important topic before anyone else – a true trailblazer.

As I mentioned in the introduction to this section, for quite a few years now the accepted wisdom was that runner's high was caused by endorphins. In fact, it's hard to believe that only a few years before that, we still had no idea about the existence of your body's own internal "morphine". For years scientists wondered why exactly was it that your brain had its own locks (opiate receptors) which morphine and other opiates (the keys) perfectly fit. Eventually endorphins (literally "endogenous morphine") were discovered as being the natural painkilling chemical produced by your body in times of stress or physical pain.

So that perfectly explains why you feel good when you exercise and why exercise treats depression right? As with anything to do with the brain, it is a little more complicated.

There is a drug called naloxone which completely neutralises the effects of opiates on the brain. If you take naloxone and then shoot heroin, you don't get high.

Which is why it is often a component of addiction treatment. It turns out that if you give someone naloxone and then they exercise, the naloxone only negates some aspects of the mood boost you get from exercise.

Subsequent research on both animals and humans has shown that exercise also increases levels of your monoamines – serotonin, dopamine and norepinephrine. Yes, exercising really is like popping a happy pill.

Exercise also improves oxygenation of the brain through improved blood flow. Your brain is a massive oxygen and energy sponge, so anything which improves delivery of this vital fuel to where it's needed is going to be hugely beneficial.

Finally, exercise also helps in an indirect way by improving the single most important aspect of brain health – sleep. Sleep is where your brain does the majority of its repair work – particularly during slow wave sleep (stage 3 & 4 "NREM" sleep) which is your deepest stage of sleep.

As you probably know, while you are asleep, your brain goes through various stages which can all be measured with a polysomnograph. You are probably most familiar with one of these stages – REM ("rapid eye movement") sleep. Slow wave sleep is when the majority of your brain's repair work happens. Exercise increases slow wave sleep, meaning that not only do you wake more refreshed than you would otherwise be, but your brain has been able to accelerate its repair work.

There is still some debate as to why exercise helps with sleep quality and quantity. I believe that it is a combination of factors. Firstly, exercise burns off a lot of stress hormones and neurotransmitters such as cortisol and norepinephrine, leading to increased relaxation and deeper sleep – you sleep much more lightly when you are stressed or physiologically aroused. Secondly, exercise, when done in the late afternoon particularly, artificially raises your core body temperature. Scientists still aren't sure why, but raising your body temperature a few hours before bed will increase slow wave sleep. This is the reason why hot baths before bed also increase slow wave sleep. The cooling that happens as your body slides down into sleep, appears to set off some kind of biochemical reaction that leads to better sleep quality.

So, if we acknowledge that exercise super-charges your brain and improves your mood, the next question is – What kind of exercise?

My philosophy is always to focus on doing what you enjoy. If you force yourself to do something you hate, you will soon give up and be back at square one. If you hate jogging, don't try to force yourself to run marathons. Be guided by how you feel. After reading so often about how jogging before breakfast accelerates weight loss, I decided to force myself to jog as soon as I woke up. It only took me a few times before I realised I hated it so much that I would never keep it up. However, come 11am each morning, I love nothing better than to hit the gym or even go for the occasional run.

Ideally you will be doing a mixture of – cardiovascular exercise, strength training and stretches. I am a massive fan of H.I.I.T (high intensity interval training) for brain health. I am also a busy, impatient guy, so I love to get my exercise done quickly. So don't think that you need to spend an hour on a treadmill. You could literally find a grassed area and do, say, 5 x 100 metre sprints and you would see massive benefits for your brain. It could be all over in 10 minutes. There is a whole new science emerging recently which supports the idea that the best kind of exercise is short in duration and high intensity.

Pick what you love and just keep at it. Remember, one of the mainstays of depression treatment is walking. Yes, just getting out of the house and walking at a leisurely pace can have a dramatic effect on symptoms of depression.

Putting it all together

Now that you have a clear understanding of all the various means with which you can modulate brain function, naturally the next question is – How do I create a plan that is right for me?

This is the juncture at which I need to reiterate a vital point – the right drug, supplement or exercise regime for you, depends on your particular circumstances. With a few exceptions (such as Omega 3, curcumin and vitamin D), there are rarely any drugs or supplements which are universally beneficial.

Let me use acetylcholine and glutamate as an example. If you are suffering from memory problems or cognitive decline, you will usually want to increase levels of acetylcholine and glutamate. However, if you are suffering from fibromyalgia or anxious depression, often you will want to tone down glutaminergic neurotransmission.

You therefore need to initially gain a clear understanding of exactly where you stand, neurologically, before you decided on a plan. Naturally it is both impossible and inadvisable for me to provide any specific recommendations – the brain is rarely black or white – however, I can provide some rough guidelines to assist you in your decision making process.

Note, that in below guidelines, it is assumed that you are already aggressively dosing Omega 3, taking a "mega B" and getting sufficient vitamin D from both sun exposure and supplementation (plus don't forget those eggs!). I am also assuming that you are doing some form of cardiovascular exercise.

As I detailed in Your Brain Electric, say for example you are depressed. Depression takes many forms and has many causes. Even if you are not depressed, some of the below may be applicable in terms of how you identify the potential cause of any mood problem or cognitive dysfunction.

Depression with low motivation

Need to - ↑ dopamine, ↑ norepinephrine, ↑ serotonin, ↓ cortisol Drugs or supplements – curcumin, alpha GPC/citicoline, rhodiola rosea

Depression with anxiety

Need to - ↑ serotonin, ↓ cortisol, ↓ norepinephrine, ↑ GABA (short term until serotonin levels increase)

Drugs or supplements – curcumin, either rhodiola rosea or St. John's Wort (would lean to St. John's Wort if you aren't taking other medication because has more of a direct action on serotonin levels), ashwagandha (for 2-3 weeks only), possibly passionflower in the evening to increase relaxation and improve sleep

Fibromyalgia

Fibromyalgia is a tricky one because it isn't a single illness, just a collection of pain and cognition-related symptoms. For example, different people get relief by –

- Modulating dopamine (using drugs such as pramipexole)

- Increasing the monoamines (using drugs such as tricyclic antidepressants or SNRIs such as duloxetine (Cymbalta)

- NMDA antagonists such as memantine or tramadol (tramadol is also an opiate and increases levels of serotonin and norepinephrine)

Therefore it is impossible to give general guidelines for fibromyalgia. However, I can give a list of drugs and supplements that have been known to be beneficial –

Duloxetine – decreases pain and improves mood-related symptoms Tramadol - decreases pain and improves mood-related symptoms

Memantine – repairs possible damage from long term glutaminergic overactivity

Tricyclics (mainly amitriptyline) - decreases pain and improves mood-related symptoms

ALCAR – improves 'brain fog'

Anxiety (without depression)

Need to - ↓ norepinephrine, ↓ dopamine, ↑ GABA, ↑ serotonin

Drugs or supplements – valerian, passionflower, 5-htp, inositol, ashwagandha

Cognitive dysfunction

Need to - ↑ dopamine, ↑ acetylcholine

Drugs or supplements – racetams, alpha GPC/citicoline, curcumin, ALCAR, alpha lipoic acid, NAC

Reading above, there is a strong chance you thought to yourself *"But hey, I am a mixture of a few of these different conditions"*. This is where the input of a doctor or nutritional expert is required on a personalised basis. There will almost always be a degree of trial and error. For example, sometimes people can start taking l- phenylalanine or l-tyrosine to improve motivation, but become too anxious. Or they can take herbal sedatives to relax at night but find they become a little depressed or sedated the following day.

Therefore, I would ask that you use this book as a starting point to assess all the range of options available. You can then use this information to provide input to your doctor or primary care provider so that the two of you can arrive at a protocol which perfectly matches your mental and neurological status.

The general list of tips for creating and maintaining a super-brain

- Get socially connected with friends and family. You only have to see this effect once to understand it. When you are feeling low or anxious, resist the urge to isolate yourself and force yourself to hang out with someone close. The mood boost is dramatic - trust me.

- Cardiovascular exercise and resistance (weight) training outperforms antidepressant medication in trial after trial. If you are not feeling up to strenuous exercise, slowly work up to it. Start with a long walk. Many doctors are now prescribing 'walking therapy' for elderly depressed patients. It seems amazing, however just going for a walk can do wonders for your mood.

- Sorry, but if you are serious about healing your brain, you need to give up alcohol until you are better. Alcohol provides a short term boost in serotonin followed by a long crash. This is one of the reasons why some people become alcoholics - they are self-medicating their depression. Certain drugs are more toxic for the brain than others. Alcohol, amphetamines (such as meth), cocaine and inhalants (such as glue sniffing) are the worst. So if you are going to start up a recreational drug habit, stick to heroin (I am joking by the way – avoid all drugs). Even marijuana, which has a benign reputation, can slowly and gradually cause all kinds of cognitive and emotional problems with long-term use. Of course, any of these drugs are not going to permanently damage your brain with one use (except maybe some inhalants), but where is the line between toxic and non-toxic? However, I am guessing that if you are reading a book like this, you either don't take drugs or you are looking to repair your brain after giving up drugs. If you are trying to repair your brain after drug addiction, take heart – the brain is an amazingly plastic organ with a surprising ability to repair years of abuse.

- Consider Cognitive Behavioral Therapy (CBT), which also regularly outperforms antidepressant medication because the beneficial changes tend to be enduring. CBT recognises that depression and anxiety are associated with faulty thinking and behaviour which perpetuates a low mood. To give an extreme example, if you lay in bed all day ruminating about how bad your life is, what kind of mood do you think you will be in? On the behavioral side, depression is often associated with avoiding certain situations or a lack of socializing. So by addressing the thinking and behaviour that is causin your depression or anxiety, you can often rebuild your brain in a healthier way.

- Learn to laugh. Engage in activities that make you laugh, such as watching comedies or playing board games with your friends.

- Create healthy sleeping habits. Deep sleep (slow wave sleep) is where your neurotransmitters are replenishes and your brain conducts its most important repair work. Avoid benzodiazepine drugs (such as Xanax, Ativan or Valium) which suppress your slow wave sleep. Unless you are sleep deprived, avoid napping during the day. Depression is associated with upset circadian rhythm and daytime naps can accentuate this problem.

- Learn to meditate. Meditation not only relaxes you and reduces the symptoms of anxiety, it also increases levels of serotonin. The other fascinating aspect of meditation involves long term changes in the brains of meditators. Scientists have known for a while that the right prefrontal cortex (PFC) tends to be more active in depressed or negative people, while the left side is associated with positive emotions. Recently, a group of scientists scanned the brains of Tibetan monks who had meditated for over 10,000 hours. They found that, compared to non-meditators, the brains of meditators had dramatically more activity in the side of the brain associated with positive emotion.

- If possible, get in the ocean. There is considerable debate as to why regular dips in the ocean appears to help with depression. Some believe that it is due to magnesium being absorbed trans-dermally, whereas others believe it is due to negative ions (negative ions are associated with positive mood). I tend to believe that the ocean is helpful because it just feels good. Cool refreshing water and the smell of the sea breeze (which has all kinds of positive connotations for most people) are the likely culprits in my opinion. If you don't live near the ocean, swimming in a pool can be just as effective for some.

Conclusion

Put simply, if you –

- Eat brain-healthy foods

- Take a range of nootropic supplements or drugs that are appropriate for you

- Treat anxiety or depression with healthy behaviours and/or antidepressant supplements or drugs

- Exercise regularly

You will be putting yourself at a huge advantage to the rest of the population. The average person doesn't know about acetylcholine and how to modulate it. The average person doesn't know all the types of foods that grow a super-brain. They let stress eat away at their brain and they rarely exercise because they are "too busy and stressed out" at work.

You have an opportunity to get an advantage over those people by being smarter about how you treat your brain. Think about it, if you are smart enough to grasp the importance of nootropics and other brain turbo-charging substances and behaviours, how smart will you be once you have put it all together?

Mind Body Soul Conclusion

If there is one thing I hope has become abundantly clear as you finish reading this book, it is that human health and happiness is a multi-faceted story. It is no use living to 100 if you are miserable in the process. Likewise, it is no use having a Ferrari-like brain if you die at 40 from heart disease or liver failure. Getting one of these wrong risks the others, or at least negates much of the benefit. And these factors all cross-communicate. Being stressed will not only make you unhappy, the elevated cortisol will wreak havoc on your body and damage your hippocampus, leading to memory deficits.

That is why I believe in the importance of bringing together my past work into this more comprehensive work.

It will also be clear that there are a range of behaviours and substances which have global effects throughout your body and brain –

- Reduce inflammation
- Consume plenty of plants in the form of vegetables (along with fruit in moderation)
- Increase consumption of omega 3 fatty acids
- Reduce sugar consumption, whether the natural fructose in fruit juices or the high fructose corn syrup in America's processed foods
- Reduce stress where possible
- Get socially connected
- Exercise regularly
- Keep your brain active

If you get just these basics right, you are 90% of the way there. Then, you can pick and choose from the other options to get the final 10%.

Good luck ☺

James Lee

May 2015

Made in the USA
Monee, IL
09 June 2022

97698813R00134